PUBLIC ENEMY NUMBER 1—STRESS

A PRACTICAL GUIDE TO THE EFFECTS OF STRESS AND NUTRITION ON THE AGING PROCESS AND LIFE EXTENSION

PUBLIC ENEMY NUMBER 1—STRESS

A PRACTICAL GUIDE TO THE EFFECTS OF STRESS AND NUTRITION ON THE AGING PROCESS AND LIFE EXTENSION

Dr. Herman Todorov Ph.D., Robert Nadler and Igor N. Todorov Ph.D.

Yorkville Press
New York, N.Y.

Editor : Patricia Aragundi
Cover Design: Norman Siegel
Interior Layout: Alberto del Rosal
Book Production: Mark Kettner

Library of Congress Catalogue-in-Publication Data

Nadler, Robert

Public Enemy Number One - Stress: A practical guide to the effects of stress and nutrition on the aging process and life extension / Herman Todorov, Robert Nadler, and I.N. Todorov.

p. cm.

Includes index.
ISBN 0-9724813-0-3
1. Stress in old age. 2. Stress (Physiology)
3. Aging - Nutritional aspects 4. Longevity - Nutritional aspects.
I. Title: Public Enemy Number One - Stress. II. Todorov, Herman III. Todorov, Igor N. IV. Title.

Yorkville Publications
919 Third Avenue Suite 2700
New York, New York 10022
Tele. 212 829-5571 Fax: 212 585-0843
E - mail: Yorkville Publications@aol.com
Website; http://www.publicenemynumber1stress.com

Printed in the United States of America

TABLE OF CONTENTS

PART I

PART II

FOREWORD

It can slowly drain the life force from your body over time or kill swiftly without warning. Yet you'll never find it on a medical chart or see it listed on a death certificate. It is called stress.

It exacts a tremendous toll on our lives. It saps our strength, robs our youth and makes us old before our time. We encounter it day in and day out, yet do little, if anything about it.

It's no wonder. In today's "pressure cooker society," the average lunch hour lasts approximately 11 minutes. Dinner is often consumed in less than 6 minutes (usually seated in front of a TV). The average workday can last 10 hours or more. We seem to be living in a society where there's virtually no quality time.

Strictly speaking, stress itself is not among the direct causes of aging, yet it plays an extremely important role in the aging process. It is an extremely powerful catalyst that causes us to age.

Readers might be surprised to find out that this book has as much to do with aging, life extension and specific measures we can take to postpone the inevitable as it does with stress. The fact is that stress and aging are inextricably bound together.

Today, the aging process is virtually no different than it was prior to the Industrial Revolution. Back then, life was considerably less hectic. Ironically, it was also considerably shorter. Nowadays, someone seventy years old is not considered old at all. The dramatic advances made in life expectancy are due in large part to antibiotics, vaccinations, cardiovascular surgery and other so-called modern medical marvels. In other words, we live longer today because we are better shielded from hardship and fatal diseases, not because we age at a slower rate. It is becoming increasingly clear that if we are to increase life expectancy in the future, we must slow down the aging process. For the first time in history, mankind has accumulated the knowledge to make this possible. To accomplish this, scientists must find ways to neutralize or postpone the many things that cause us to grow old.

There are two more important points we would like to make before we go on. Chances are you think of stress as a state of mind. However, it is also a chemical state of the body. A person can be perfectly at rest and yet still be in a state of chronic stress in terms of body chemistry. Secondly, the steps we take to slow down the aging process can be effective only if we keep stress in check.

Another subject we will explore in this book is nutrition. An intelligent, well-balanced diet can go a long way toward providing you with the kind of good health required to take full advantage of a longer life span. Conversely, neglect proper nutrition and you diminish all other steps you take towards life extension.

This book is divided into three parts. The first part is a comprehensive review of our current body of knowledge on modern anti-aging science. It provides a more thorough explanation of the mechanisms of aging and how to counteract them.

Readers interested in the more practical applications may find it profitable to jump directly to the second and third parts. The second part focuses on the relationship between aging and stress. The third focuses on the everyday things you can do to ensure that you add more life to your years as well as more years to your life.

For those readers, the first section can be used as reference whenever their understanding of fundamental science or some practical recommendation requires further clarification.

Living to a ripe old age is no accident. It is a lifelong pursuit that starts when we are young and doesn't end until we've drawn our last breath. It's something we must work at constantly.

This book was written in the hope of providing you with the tools to help build your own personal life extension program. We will cover the factors that determine why we age and at what rate. We will detail the effects of aging on our bodies and our minds - how aging affects our ability to function, adapt and flourish - even how it affects our sex lives.

Needless to say, understanding the true scope and magnitude of the aging process takes years of study. However by the time you finish this book , we believe you'll be equipped to prolong and enhance

this book , we believe you'll be equipped to prolong and enhance your life.

Perhaps someday the world will be free of age-related diseases. Maybe in the not-too-distant future the average life will span more than a century. There may come a time when cancer, heart disease and other life-threatening conditions cease to exist.

We can't say when, but that day is coming. However, for you that day may be close at hand the moment you turn this page.

PART I

CHAPTER 1

AGING – POSTPONING THE INEVITABLE.

You won't find the definition of aging in most dictionaries. The closest you may come to it is the verb *"to age"* which means to grow old. While this definition is vague and of little use, we do have a reasonable understanding of what aging is all about. It is the seemingly endless process of wearing down, impairing and eventually sapping the life force of all living things. This is certainly true, but it represents only a small part of a much larger picture.

Obviously, no organism is immune to aging. However, we age quite differently, at different rates and in somewhat different ways. For instance, among similar species like mammals, the rate of aging may differ drastically from one species to another. Even among human beings, the age of individuals who die of natural causes varies within an extremely wide range. Given this, why does one person remain vibrant and filled with life at ninety and yet another in his fifties appear drained and afflicted with a host of diseases? Uncovering the answers to these questions not only holds the key to understanding the nature of aging, but also the key to increasing life expectancy.

Scientists define aging as a process that increases the probability of death with time. Again, that's hard to argue with, but it adds little to our body of knowledge. What's more, it is now evident that aging is not one single process, but a group of complicated interdependent processes affecting every facet of an organism's life cycle.

A comprehensive understanding of aging requires familiarity with all of its integral components. In this section, we will attempt to provide you with a concise, yet reasonably complete picture, of what today's science knows about the aging process. You see, we firmly believe that someone who embarks on a life extension journey should at the very least, have a general understanding of the nature of aging.

While life can be cut short by a drunk driver or some other twist of fate, longevity is by no means an accident. Luck does play a role in that you may be fortunate enough to inherit genes that increase your chances of a longer life. However, there are no guarantees. How long you live depends on a thoughtful, continuous program directed toward life extension. Unfortunately, clean living and a healthy lifestyle can onlytake you so far. When you let nature run its course, what you get is a "natural" life expectancy of seventy to eighty years. In fact, even this is almost twice the natural length of human life prior to the Industrial Revolution.

Remarkable advances in relation to increasing life expectancy have occurred in the Twentieth century. These were mostly due to the conquering of infectious diseases with antibiotics, improved sanitation and public health practices, better living and working conditions and other medical, technological and social breakthroughs. There is nothing "natural" about many of these things, yet we accept them because they work to our advantage. It seems, however, that the present methodology of increasing life expectancy has largely been exhausted.

When the next steps in life extension come, there's a good chance they will come from uncovering the biological mechanisms of aging and finding ways to negate them. In fact, we've already made tremendous strides toward this goal. Several anti-aging approaches have been developed. For instance, with our current knowledge, we can double the life span of laboratory animals. Of course, it would be naive to expect the same dramatic results in humans, yet it's safe to say that many of the methods that work in mice should have relatively similar effects in human beings because of a high degree of biochemical similarity. Again, these methods are not natural in the strict sense, because they disrupt the fate of the organism. We do not need to focus on prescription drugs as tools for life extension. Although a few drugs have shown promise in this regard. Most are expensive, not readily available and have a relatively high level of toxicity. At present, using prescription drugs for life extension is neither reasonable nor realistic for a vast majority of the population. The life extension strategy detailed in the third part of this book is mainly based on the natural substances normally found in animal or plant tissues. However, the amounts required for significant life extension cannot always be readily obtained by maintaining a balanced diet alone.

Over the past few decades we have seen tremendous growth in understanding the nature of aging. Aging is associated with a gradual decline in the functional capacity of the organs and systems of the body, all of which result in the loss of adaptability to both internal and external stimuli. As an organism ages, smaller and smaller incidents become greater and greater threats to survival. In the elderly, even a relatively minor stress, like the flu, can result in death.

We have grown accustomed to thinking of our bodies as being constant and stable. This couldn't be further from the truth. Our bodies are chemical mini-reactors, with energy and matter constantly flowing in and out, and billions of molecular transformations occurring every second. As long as we are alive, our bodies are in a state of equilibrium. Each of our organ systems work constantly to maintain this incredibly delicate balance. Some cells die, others divide; damaged molecules are constantly being repaired or replaced. Although the mechanisms of self-repair are remarkably efficient, some damage is irreprable and cumulative over time. The rate of aging is largely dependent on the rate of accumulation of unrepaired lesions and the efficiency of both repair and replacement mechanisms. Irreversible damage to key molecular structures occurs throughout all stages of life, so it is never too early to take steps toward ensuring a healthy life extension program. In fact, it is important to get a good head start. After all, damage accumulates more rapidly with age because repair mechanisms lose their efficiency.

All systems of an organism deteriorate with age, but the rate of decline varies markedly among these systems. A person may succumb to pneumonia due to a weak immune system even though other systems are in perfect working order. A comprehensive anti-aging approach should support all vital systems. There is little solace in having excellent lungs, youthful skin and 20/20 vision if you have just suffered a fatal heart attack. Fortunately, many nutritional and lifestyle measures that benefit one system of the body often strengthen others. A good example are the nutrients that benefit several body systems simultaneously, like antioxidants such as vitamins A, C, E, selenium, amino acid cysteine, coenzyme Q-10 and lipoic acid.

Aging may manifest itself simply as a functional decline of organs and tissue, but more often it shows itself as **age-related** or **degenerative diseases**. The risk of these diseases increases dramatically with age. Notably, all higher organisms, especially mammals, have similar age-related diseases, indicating the similarity between their aging mechanisms. Hence, whatever extends life in animals has a chance of working in humans. Age-related diseases include atherosclerosis (clogged arteries leading to heart attacks and stroke), hypertension, diabetes, cancer, immune disturbances, depression, osteoporosis (fragile bones), Alzheimer's disease, Parkinson's disease, cataracts, and other maladies. In developed countries, age-related diseases account for over 80% of all deaths. On the other hand, life extension methods help prevent and can even reverse age-related diseases. Comprehensive life extension can not only increase the years between the dates on one's tombstone, but improve the quality of life enjoyed between them.

Stress — A major key to aging

Stress is closely tied to age-related diseases as well as to the aging process itself. Part II of this book is largely devoted to this subject. As a result, we will discuss here briefly, stress, or more accurately, the **stress response.** The stress response is essentially a complex adaptive reaction of an organism that is vital to its survival, especially during injuries, infections or immediate dangers. The stress response was especially important in the early days of man when life was tennuous and danger, infections and struggle were part of daily life. Stress triggers quick mobilization of energy reserves, which are routed to the organs vital to immediate survival, particularly the brain, heart and muscles. In essence, the stress response is a "biological overdrive" mechanism which helps us escape potential harm, but not without a great deal of wear and tear on the body. It is imperative that we have a good stress response. If the stress response in an emergency is too weak, the organism either dies or suffers additional damage which often manifests itself in diseases and accelerated aging. If the stress response is excessive or prolonged, it becomes a damaging force itself. Numerous studies in animals have shown that an optimal stress response is one of the key elements of longevity. As we age, we gradually lose the capacity for an optimal stress response and our bodies become less able to adapt to adversity. Loss of stress resistance accelerates aging, which, in turn, further disrupts our ability to adapt to adversity. This vicious cycle is a major factor in the aging process and development of age-related diseases. Fortunately, the cycle can be broken or at least slowed, as you will soon see.

THE EVOLUTION OF AGING

Biology students often wonder why there are so few long-lived species. After all, aren't the basic principles of evolution the same for most organisms? All species use the same information carriers (DNA and RNA) and similar building blocks for their cells (amino acids, proteins, lipids, etc.). Although Darwin's evolutionary theory is often treated as yesterday's news, it remains one of the best tools for understanding the differences among species. Only those species survive that adapt to the environment by developing advantageous traits. Long life is obviously a great bonus for the individual, but in many cases it does not provide any competitive advantage to a species and in some cases may actually be a disadvantage. Imagine a situation in which the environment constantly changes, at least a little. To remain competitive, a species would also have to change constantly. Living organisms evolve through spontaneous mutations which are random changes in the genetic blueprint (DNA). A species evolution is affected only by the mutations in germ cells (cells involved in reproduction, such as sperm and eggs) because only these are passed on to the progeny. Most mutations can be harmful or even lethal.

In a constantly changing environment, a faster rate of reproduction is advantageous because there are more opportunities for producing mutations that are better adapted for new conditions. These better-adapted mutations will survive and reproduce. The need for such rapid turnover does not favor long-lived organisms because they tend to be slower in reaching the reproductive stage in the life cycle. Young reproductive members of a species are forced to compete for resources with their long lived counterparts. The superefficient self-repair mechanism required for longer life consumes resources that might otherwise be used for reproduction. Nonetheless, long-living species do evolve and we are the prime example.

There seem to be several evolutionary reasons why **homo sapiens** live longer than other mammals. An advanced, highly-developed brain gives man enormous advantages. For an individual to develop to full potential takes years, and having parents around to nurture and teach. The payback, in evolutionary terms, is worth the cost because an offspring with a powerful brain has a greater ability of survival. Our larger brain also helps compensate for adverse changes in the environment by creating artificial habitats, devising new methods for food production, etc. As opposed to other species, humans do not need to undergo further evolutionary changes to survive in a changing environment: they simply create their own. Humans can afford and even benefit from relatively slow reproduction and long life. The downside of this is the lack of evolutionary pressure on humans to evolve toward an even longer life span. Fortunately, that powerful brain of ours can help us take matters into our own hands.

CHAPTER 2

THEORIES OF AGING COME OF AGE.

Aging is not one single process. It is a group of processes involving many different mechanisms, each contributing its own distinct signature to the process. Perhaps that's why there are several theories of aging, each addressing some aspect of the aging process. Yet none of which seem to provide a complete picture.

Aging is such a vast, complicated subject that it's difficult to grasp in its entirety. Despite this, we feel that we can provide you with a good overall picture that will not only help you understand aging, but also suggest ways to retard the process.

To begin with, the mechanisms of aging can be roughly divided into two groups: (1) the accumulation of random damage, or **microaccidents**; and (2) genetic programs, or **aging clocks**.

The first group includes various types of random events that damage vital structures in the organism. For example, free radicals - highly reactive by-products of normal cellular respiration can randomly damage the key molecules of life (DNA, proteins and lipids). Cell membranes are especially susceptible to free radical attacks because they are rich in highly reactive unsaturated fatty acids. **Mutagens** - chemicals that have the capacity to genetically alter DNA - can disturb the normal function of genes. Some reactive chemicals, such as aldehydes, can tie together *(cross-link)* cellular components, reducing their mobility and functional capacity. Some of these offenders, such as UV-rays radiation or toxic pollutants are environmental in nature and can be avoided. Most of the damage, however, comes from substances generated within our cells and part of our normal physiology. These things are inescapable.

Harmful molecular accidents occur in our cells constantly. Most are harmless because the damage is repaired quickly by reparation enzymes. But a small percentage of lesions are missed and the damage that remains is irreverseable. The accumulation of damage accelerates with age, partly because the repair mechanisms become damaged and lose efficiency. It is also conceivable, though unproven, that some repair mechanisms may be shut down by the genetic programs of aging.

Back when aging research was in its infancy, there raged a heated debate over the existence of aging clocks. Today, we know that most single cell organisms and some primitive species do not have them. There is now conclusive evidence that complex organisms such as mammals have not one aging clock, but several.

Two of these aging clocks are of particular importance: **the central aging clock** and **the cellular aging clock**. The central aging clock is located in the brain and plays a critical role in both the development and aging of an organism. Cellular aging clocks are in almost every cell in our bodies and limit the number of divisions a cell can undergo.

Other types of aging clocks include the clock that controls the reproductive function in women and male pattern hair loss. However, it would appear that these secondary clocks are at least somewhat dependent on the rate of the central aging clock and cellular clocks.

Biological clocks, especially the ones that affect aging, are not really clocks in the true sense. Their pace can vary markedly among individuals and even more so among species; different events cause these clocks to speed up or slow down. Stress and possibly overeating tend to speed up aging clocks. Stress reduction and nutrients that revitalize certain brain structures, such as the **hypothalamus** and **pituitary glands**, slow down these clocks. In rodents, severe caloric restriction before sexual maturation leads to a two-fold increase in life span.

Unfortunately, this highly effective method only works in rodents, not primates. For humans severe caloric restriction initiated early in life can cause brain damage and shorten life expectancy. Statistics indicate that maintaining close to ideal weight is of primary importance for increased life expectancy in humans.

Free radicals

With the possible exception of money, too much of anything can have a disastrous effect on life. Take freedom, for example. It is wonderful when exercised within the framework of laws - laws that protect our lives, our rights and our property. Without these laws, people would be free to do whatever they please - including harming their neighbors and society at large. In other words, freedom without restraint can wreak havoc.

If you take the idea of freedom in society and apply it to free radicals, you may find intriguing similarities. Free radicals are highly reactive chemicals. Most chemicals in the body interact with each other relatively slowly and within certain predetermined patterns called **metabolic pathways**. These patterns or rules are enforced by special proteins called **enzymes** that facilitate and guide chemical reactions.

However, with free radicals, it's a whole other story. They tend to react quickly and indiscriminately with whatever cellular structures are at hand, inflicting damage as they go.

Like death and taxes, free radicals are an inevitable consequence of life. All higher organisms generate energy by slowly burning (oxidizing) fuel: carbohydrates, fats and protein. This energy is generated in a kind of **biological microreactor** called mitochondria and the energy produced is stored in the form of ATP, which is a form of universal biological energy (**currency**). This nifty little power-generating enterprise also produces highly toxic by-products, a.k.a. free radicals. For as long as we breathe, free radicals will remain a part of us.

Free radicals can react with essentially any structure within the cell. Cell membranes are especially vulnerable because they contain unsaturated fatty acids that are highly reactive. Free radicals make membranes rigid, fragile and leaky. A cell with this type of membrane cannot function properly or may possibly rupture and die. DNA also suffers from free radical damage and free radicals may damage vital genes or cause cells to turn cancerous.

During the course of evolution, organisms developed the means to protect themselves against free radical damage. Several enzymes that help neutralize the effects and their derivatives are **superoxide dismutase** (SOD, neutralizes the superoxide radical), **catalase** (inactivates hydrogen peroxide) and **glutathione peroxidase** (participates in neutralizing lipid and other peroxides). Cells are also protected by various antioxidants (free radical scavengers) including vitamins C, E, coenzyme-Q10, selenium, glutathione and melatonin. Despite this incredibly complex security system, a few free radicals continually manage to escape and cause damage. As stress, malnutrition, old age or illness diminish the body's defenses, the damage tends to be greater.

The idea that free radicals have an impact on the aging process was first proposed by Dr. Denham Harman in the mid-Fifties. For many years it was considered a curious and far-fetched hypothesis. However, in the past two decades, scientists have accumulated enough evidence to openly embrace this theory. Today, it has become one of the most widely accepted and well-documented theories on aging.

The amount of free radical damage appears to be directly proportionate to the organism's metabolic rate (the rate at which calories are burned). The metabolic rate of a rat is about 7 times that of a human. It is estimated that rats suffer about 100,000 free radical "hits" to DNA per cell, and humans only about 10,000 or so. This is probably why humans have a much longer life span than rats. In fact, when the metabolic rate of rats is lowered by severe food restriction, their life span increases dramatically.

Each cell has two parts, the **nucleus** and **mitochondria**, both containing DNA: The nucleus contains most of the cell's genetic material packed into chromosomes; mitochondria contain a very small, but indispensable portion of cellular DNA. As it turns out, free radical damage to DNA is much greater in mitochondria than in the nucleus. The DNA from rat mitochondria has about 10 times more free radical damage than does DNA from the nucleus of the same tissue. This is because most free radicals are formed in mitochondria where the fuel is burned. Besides, mitochondrial DNA isn't as well protected by proteins and repair systems as found in nuclear DNA. As time passes, the energy producing capacity of mitochondria dwindles. As a result, mitochondria are the first cellular system to degenerate with age. As a result, cells become less active metabolically, leading to decreased functionality of organs, poor adaptability and progression of degenerative diseases.

Stress also appears to be a major contributor to the burnout of mitochondria. Stress makes mitochondria work harder by raising energy demands, which leads in turn, to more oxidative by-products - free radicals. During prolonged or intensive stress, mitochondrial membranes can become so damaged by free radicals that they leak, disrupting energy production and perpetuate even more destruction. This results in disproportionately severe oxidative damage, which is thought to accelerate aging and promote disease.

The fact that mitochondria are particularly susceptible to free radical damage makes them a potential target for anti-aging and anti-stress intervention. Certain nutrients have been shown to improve mitochondrial function: acetyl-L-carnitine (ALC) and coenzyme Q10 (CoQ10). ALC is part of the mechanism for the transport of fatty acids into the mitochondria. Although it can be synthesized in the body, the rate of synthesis decreases with age. Supplementation with ALC speeds up the utilization of fats by mitochondria, improving energy production. Several studies have shown ALC to lower cholesterol levels, increase HDL and improve cardiovascular and brain function.

CoQ10 has two important roles: it is the core of the cellular respiratory system located in the mitochondria and it is an antioxidant. CoQ10 improves both the rate and efficiency of energy production and, at the same time protects mitochondria from free radical damage. The body can produce CoQ10, but many factors, including age, illness, cholesterol-level and malnutrition, can impair production. CoQ10 is sometimes called a "biomarker of aging", because its level correlates directly with aging and degenerative diseases. In one study,

CoQ10 supplementation increased life expectancy in mice by 50%. A large number of studies clearly demonstrate the efficiency of CoQ10 in combating congestive heart failure and other diseases related to heart muscle. Other conditions that appear to be helped by CoQ10 include hypertension, decreased immunity and muscular atrophy.

There is quite a body of evidence that free radical damage accumulates with age. For instance, a two-year-old rat has twice the number of oxidative lesions (lesions caused by oxygen free radicals) in DNA than does a young rodent. The frequency of mutations in lymphocytes of elderly people is about 9 times greater than in the lymphocytes of babies. Werner syndrome and progeria, two diseases that cause dramatically accelerated aging, are associated with a marked increase in free radical damage.

Recent studies clarifying long-lived mutations in various species provided remarkable insights into the link between aging and free radicals. It was found that mutations that knock out a single gene (called age-1) i.e., a species of worm **Caenorhabditis elegans,** produced a 70% increase in life span. It turned out that mutant worms had increased levels of two key free radical scavenging enzymes, superoxide dismutase and catalase and it was suggested that the gene knocked out by these mutations encodes an inhibitor of antioxidant systems of the cell. In another study, researchers used selective breeding to produce fruit flies (Drosophila Melanogaster) that enjoyed twice the normal life span. One important difference between regular and long-lived flies was a higher activity of superoxide dismutase in the latter.

In the pioneering days of radiobiology, a field of science concerned with the biological effects of radiation, researchers encountered a puzzling phenomenon. Low-level radiation treatments protected animals from higher exposures as well as many from other stresses, such as mutagens, toxins and oxidants. Later, it was found that a mild, temporary increase in free radical formation caused by radiation stimulates the production of various free radical scavenging enzymes, improving resistance to future damage.

Needless to say, moving next door to a nuclear power plant to acquire better stress resistance is not highly recommended. However, there is a much simpler solution guaranteed to make your cheeks glow, not your spleen. Exercise. It is also a mild-to-moderate free radical inducer. This stands to reason: the more fuel you burn, the more oxidative by-products you accumulate. A reasonable amount of periodic exercise will stimulate your own antioxidant defenses which remain enhanced long after exercise. On the other hand, excessive exercise, which is a severe physical stress, can overwhelm your protective systems and accelerate aging. With exercise, there can be too much of a good thing (unless you are a professional athlete with a multi-million dollar shoe contract).

Diet, like exercise, is another very important part of maintaining good antioxidant defenses. A balanced diet provides the building blocks for the body's free radicals defenses. Vitamins A, C, E are antioxidants and the amino acid cysteine is a component of **glutathione**, a crucial intracellular antioxidant; copper, zinc and manganese are needed for the proper function of superoxide dismutase, and selenium - for glutathione peroxidase (both are key free radical scavenging enzymes). Fruits and vegetables contain a wide variety of natural antioxidants including numerous flavonoids, **carotenoids** and **anthocyanins**. It appears that natural antioxidants vary in their affinity for different types of cells or parts of the cell, as well as in their effectiveness against specific types of free radicals. A diet with plenty of fruits and vegetables seems to provide the best all-round antioxidant protection. Many studies have demonstrated that such a diet reduces the risk of degenerative diseases. Current guidelines of the National Cancer Institute and National Academy of Sciences suggest eating at least 2-4 servings of fruit and 3-5 servings of vegetables a day.

Even though a balanced diet high in fruits and vegetables is important for longevity, it appears that additional antioxidant supplements may provide additional benefits.

Central clock

Does the human body have a central clock that paces the aging of all its systems? The answer is simple: yes and no. For a comedian that's a punch line. But in this case there is logic behind this seemingly illogical answer. On one hand, it appears that we humans don't have a specific central program whose sole purpose is aging. On the other, we definitely do have a program of development, i.e., a program that makes a single cell (*zygote*) develop into a complex organism. Some of the mechanisms of this development program seem to lack an "off" switch and continue to run long after the organism's development is complete. These mechanisms are essential during growth and sexual maturation, but they appear to have an array of late side effects. In fact, these mechanisms become harmful in a mature organism because they act as if development were still in progress. The result is accelerated aging and the potential onset of degenerative diseases. In other words, the central aging clock appears to be a function of our developmental program that doesn't switch off after its job is done.

This approach to the central aging clock is the basis behind the neuroendocrine theory of aging developed by a remarkable Russian scientist, Dr. Vladimir Dilman. Neuroendocrine theory has to do with the interaction of the central nervous system and the endocrine system (the endocrine system regulates body functions through hormones). For simplicity's sake we'll refer to Dilman's theory as the central aging clock theory. The theory was first proposed in the 1950's, when it was little more than an educated guess. However, in the last fifty years, it has stood up to almost every challenge proposed by the scientific community.

To understand the central aging clock theory, we must first under stand **homeostasis**. Basically, homeostasis is the proper balance of an organism's internal environment. For the body to function normally, key physiological parameters must be maintained within a certain range: the temperature should be about 37°C (98.6°F), blood pressure about 120/80, blood sugar 70-120 mg/dl, etc. In other words, the body must maintain its homeostasis. If homeostasis is disturbed, the body uses every available means to restore its balance. Failure to do so can result in death.

The tricky part is that a newborn's homeostasis is different from that of an older child, both of which are different from an adult. For instance, the average level of hemoglobin (a molecule that transports oxygen in the blood) in infant boys is about 11 mg/100 ml, in ten-year-old boys about 13 mg/100 ml, and in adult men, 15 mg/100 ml; the average blood pressure in ten year olds is about 100/60 and in young adults - 120/80. On one hand, an organism has to maintain homeostasis relevant to that particular stage of development. On the other hand, the organism has to change or shift its homeostasis to ultimately reach the parameters necessary for maturity.

That's exactly what our developmental program does - it gradually shifts homeostasis, "pushing" the body to consume and expend more energy, increase in size and develop reproductive organs - in other words, to grow and mature. Unfortunately, these gradual changes do not stop completely once an organism reaches maturity. They continue throughout its entire life. So growth and development stop at some point, but the driving mechanisms don't. The program continues to run, but now it does damage rather than good, contributing to aging and age-related diseases.

Why haven't we developed an off-switch for our developmental program to prevent it causing accelerated aging in later life? Apparently, such an off-switch was not important to the species' survival. Whatever the evolutionary reason, we have the equivalent of a built-in central aging clock. Fortunately, biological clocks are not rigid and their pace can be altered. Some influences will speed up the central aging clock while others slow it down.

Before discussing how to slow down this clock, we should really describe its basic mechanism. The "central computer" largely responsible for the body's homeostasis is the area of the brain called the hypothalamus. The hypothalamus works as a control mechanism that constantly monitors dozens of the body's internal parameters. If any parameter moves out of range, the hypothalamus sends a signal to the pituitary gland which controls the endocrine system. Using a corporate management chart as a metaphor, if the hypothalamus represents the board of directors in regard to homeostasis, the pituitary represents the CEO. The pituitary translates the signals from the hypothalamus into a hormonal message to the peripheral endocrine glands, such as the thyroid or adrenals "management". In turn, peripheral endocrine glands use their own hormones to give instructions to the work force - target organs and tissues. In most cases, the instructions are to increase or decrease some physiological function.

Another important concept worthy of discussion here is negative feedback, a.k.a. **feedback inhibition**. For example, in winter the body needs to raise its metabolic rate to compensate for colder weather. The hypothalamus sends the appropriate signal to the pituitary, which sends a signal to the thyroid to secrete more thyroxin (the hormone that raises metabolic rate). The resulting rise in thyroxin is sensed by the hypothalamus, which then stops sending the initial signal. Essentially this is an example of negative feedback. It is the ability of the system to discontinue an initial stimulatory signal after a certain goal has been attained.

As previously mentioned, the body's development requires gradual shifts in homeostasis. The hypothalamus is the driving force behind this shift. The neuroendocrine theory of aging proposes that the hypothalamus implements the organism's development program (which later becomes the aging clock) by becoming less responsive to negative feedback. For instance, the ovaries in young girls produce only small amounts of estrogens, but enough to exert negative feedback; i.e., to make the hypothalamus stop urging the production of more estrogen. With increasing age, the hypothalamus becomes less responsive to negative feedback and stimulates the ovaries to produce more estrogen. This leads to a well-known rise in estrogen levels which eventually leads to sexual maturation. Similar shifts of homeostasis occur during development in all body systems. Unfortunately, after maturity hypothalamic responses to negative feedback continue to decrease. This inspires further homeostatic shifts, which now produce a negative effect, contributing to aging and degenerative diseases.

So, how do these homeostatic shifts cause aging and age-related diseases? A number of interrelated mechanisms seem to be involved in this process. However, putting them under the proverbial microscope would still leave us nowhere. The most important of these include age-related insulin excess (hyperinsulinemia), decreased carbohydrate tolerance, abnormal adaptive response, age-related depression and increased secretion of gonadotropins (hormones that stimulate the activity of sex glands).

Age-related insulin excess and decreased carbohydrate tolerance are homeostatic shifts that have to do with energy utilization. Insulin is a hormone secreted by the pancreas in response to the rise in blood sugar (glucose), normally occurring after a meal. Insulin promotes the transport of glucose, amino acids and fats into cells, where they are either consumed as energy, stored or used as structural material. The typical scenario after eating goes something like this: as food is digested and absorbed, blood glucose rises, triggering the secretion of insulin which in an hour or so brings blood glucose to its original level or even lower. With age, the ability of muscle and other tissue to absorb glucose in response to insulin decreases while the amount of insulin secreted after a meal increases. The net effect is that we have higher blood glucose for a longer period of time and more circulating insulin in the bloodstream. There has been much controversy over whether decreased sensitivity of muscle to insulin causes excessive insulin secretion or vice versa. According to the neuroendocrine theory of aging, both are caused, at least to some degree, by the central hypothalamic clock. The mechanism by which the hypothalamus causes these shifts appears to be complex and involves subtle changes in the appetite center to glucose and altered regulation of growth hormone secretion.

Excess insulin and decreased glucose tolerance raise the levels of cholesterol, LDL and triglycerides, promote cell damage through the processes of glycation and cross-linking, causing sodium retention and numerous other disruptions. As a result, these metabolic shifts contribute to the development of most age-related diseases including atherosclerosis, hypertension, diabetes, upper body obesity, impaired immunity and increased risk of cancer.

The most common example of extreme glucose intolerance is non-insulin dependent diabetes (type II diabetes). Patients with this condition have high blood sugar despite being able to produce insulin. In fact, in the initial stage of type II diabetes, the levels of insulin are often above normal. Untreated diabetes produces numerous complications, many of which can be considered as an acceleration of aging and degenerative diseases.

Glucose tolerance can be improved and insulin excess reduced. A diet low in fiber and high in saturated fat, overeating and chromium deficiency can produce excess insulin. Moderate exercise, weight loss, and a diet low in saturated fat and high in fiber, can help reduce insulin excess.

Another grave consequence of the central aging clock is the change in the body's response to stress as we grow older. During stress, the hypothalmus issues an "order" to produce stress steroids, the hormones that mediate many of the effects of stress on the body. When the level of stress steroids in the blood rise, the hypothalmus senses it and sends an "order" to stop production, allowing a return to normal levels. As the central aging clock continues to tick, the hypothalmus gradually loses this ability. As a result, the hypothalmus will often "fire up" some hormone and then turn it off. Some older people produce too many stress steroids, even in a total state of rest. These individuals live in a state of chronic stress without ever suspecting it.

As most people have learned from experience, stress may inflict damage on any part of the body. The hypothalmus is no exception. But stress-induced damage to the hypothalmus and related brain structures has a really nasty consequence - it speeds up the central aging clock. In fact, there appears to be a vicious cycle: the central aging clock gradually disturbs the body's normal response to stress which, in turn, accelerates the aging clock itself.

According to the neuroendocrine theory, insulin excess, impaired carbohydrate tolerance and abnormal stress are the major contributors to aging and degenerative diseases. There are, however, many other ways in which the central aging clock appears to contribute to age-related problems. For instance, the hypothalamus is probably responsible for the gradual increase in the levels of prolactin. This hormone is secreted by the pituitary gland and stimulates milk production in women. The role of prolactin in men is unclear, but it is well established that a high prolactin level contributes to the development of benign prostate enlargement (a condition almost ubiquitous in elderly men) and raises the risk of impotence.

It would appear that the best way to slow down the central aging clock is to improve the responsiveness of the hypothalamus to negative feedback and the rest of the body systems. Evidence indicates that the levels of neurotransmitters (chemicals that carry messages between brain cells) in the hypothalamus are directly related to its

Central aging clock is accelerated by:	Central aging clock is slowed down by:
Stress; abnormal response to stress	Improving stress resistance; restoration of optimal response to stress; avoidance of intense or prolonged stress
Overeating; excess calories	Caloric restriction (in rodents), maintenance of ideal body weight (in humans)
Impaired glucose/carbohydrate tolerance	Improved glucose/carbohydrate tolerance
Insulin excess	Optimal insulin release
Depression; decreased neurotransmitter levels in the hypothalamus	Optimal emotional state; elevation of neurotransmitter levels in the hypothalamus
Lack of melatonin and other pineal gland hormones	Restoration of the levels of melatonin and other pineal gland hormones prevention of free radical damage to the brain
Free radical damage to the brain due to oxidation, ionizing radiation or environmental toxins	

Table 1. Factors believed to speed up or slow down the central aging clock located in the hypothalamus and related brain structures.

responsiveness to negative feedback. The factors believed to slow down aging also tend to raise the level of neurotransmitters in the hypothalamus. More importantly, whatever raises the neurotransmitter levels in the hypothalamus tends to slow down the aging clock. There are many other factors that affect the central aging clock, but we'll discuss most of them in detail in future chapters.

THE CELLULAR CLOCK

Bacteria are immortal, at least in theory. A bacterial cell placed in favorable conditions will grow and divide indefinitely. For the better part of this century, it was thought that cells from higher species were also immortal, capable of dividing indefinitely under proper conditions. In 1912, Alexis Carrel, then at the Rockefeller Institute, started an experiment to test how long chicken fibroblasts could divide. Fibroblasts are connective tissue cells whose job is to build the resilient three-dimensional framework that supports other cells. Carrel fed the fibroblasts with a special broth derived from chicken embryos, supplying fresh broth every few days. Excess cells were periodically discarded. The fibroblasts continued dividing year after year, without any signs of slowing down. After Carrel's death some thirty years later, the experiment was stopped. It seemed that in a proper environment the cells of higher organisms were as immortal as bacteria.

In the early 1960's, Leonard Hayflick made an observation that put an end to Carrel's theory once and for all. Hayflick found that human fibroblasts in culture would divide about 50 times and then stop. It appeared that Carrel's experimental technique had a flaw. The nourishing broth he used to feed his fibroblasts was likely to have contained a small number of fibroblasts, so new cells were apparently added every few days. The maximal number of divisions the cells could undergo in culture became known as the Hayflick Limit.

It has been suggested that the Hayflick Limit is in fact, a genetic program that prevents cell division after a given number of cycles.

Why would our cells need to have such a program? The current view is that a built-in limit on the number of possible cell divisions reduces the risk of uncontrolled cell growth resulting in cancer. Indeed, studies indicate that the genetic clock in cancer cells is broken, allowing them to grow indefinitely.

Research over the past few years has provided an intriguing insight into possible molecular mechanisms, defining the Hayflick limit in cancer cells. In the cells of higher organisms, chromosomes are capped with special DNA structures called **telomeres**. The main role of telomeres is to protect the ends of chromosomes from degradation. During cell division, the chromosomes are duplicated through the process of DNA replication (copying). However, due to the nature of this process, the extreme ends of the telomeres cannot be copied. Picture a road-laying machine that can only move while it is on the road. When it has reached the end of that road, there is a new layer of asphalt over the entire road behind it except for the spot under the machine. To cover the remaining spot, the machine must move past it, but it can't because it is at the end of the road. A similar scenario occurs during chromosome replication, thus, the very end of each telomere is never copied, which leads to progressively shortening telomeres with each cell division. After its telomeres have shortened beyond a certain point, the cell loses its ability to divide (This doesn't occur in bacteria because their chromosomes are circular and do not have telomeres). When fibroblasts approach the 50th division they begin to look old, their metabolic activity decreases, they increase in size, and accumulate lipofuscin, the pigment responsible for age spots.

Could it be that aging is the result of the cell's inability to divide once it has reached the Hayflick Limit? Like most other questions in this chapter, this one has no straight answer. It appears that in some tissues, such as the skin and the lining of blood vessels, the Hayflick Limit may indeed be a part of the aging mechanism. For instance, the acceleration of atherosclerosis with age may in part, result from the reduced ability of vascular epithelial cells to divide. Age-related loss of skin moisture and elasticity may also be associated with the Hayflick Limit. On the other hand, most cells in the brain, retina, nerves and muscles normally do not divide and probably never even approach the "allowed" number of divisions.

Can the Hayflick Limit be overridden? Unfortunately, the answer is yes. Some mutations seen in cancer cells do exactly that as well as some viruses, most notably the papilloma virus, which immortalize the cells they infect. At least one cellular mechanism for overriding the Hayflick limit has actually been found. All cells appear to have the gene that encodes an enzyme (called telomerase) capable of restoring shortened telomeres. The cells in which telomerase are active seem to be immortal. In most normal cells, however, the activity of telomerase is somehow suppressed so they cannot divide beyond the limit.

What does all this mean in terms of life extension? First, the existence of the Hayflick Limit may contribute to age-related changes and diseases in some tissues such as the skin and blood vessels. Second, even if we could, it may be dangerous to completely abolish the Hayflick limit because of the increased likelihood of cancer. And third, it appears that the number of divisions before a cell reaches its limit is not carved in stone. Different environmental factors may accelerate or slow down the cellular clock. Increased free radical formation has been shown to shorten the Hayflick limit and some growth factors (proteins that stimulate cell growth) were found to extend it in some tissue. An intriguing result was obtained recently by a group of Dutch scientists who demonstrated that garlic extract could extend the Hayflick Limit and improve the function of skin fibroblasts in culture. A group of scientists at Geron, a biotechnology company, have inserted a working copy of the telomerase gene in fibroblasts with the result that the cells have exceeded the Hayflick limit without showing any signs of senescence, remaining young and robust and are still "happily" dividing.

What can we do to minimize the contribution of the cellular clock to the overall aging process? It may be possible in the near future to use genetic engineering to change the program responsible for the Hayflick Limit (although this may produce more problems than it solves like increasing the risk of cancer). The best we can do for now is to avoid unnecessary cell divisions and, possibly, to extend the limit by improving the internal environment of our bodies. Avoiding unnecessary cell divisions means minimizing exposure to the factors that promote it. Most agents that damage cells also promote cell division, indirectly - in particular, free radicals, inflammation, mutagens, some toxins and UV-radiation. Antioxidants appear to have the opposite effect. Some substances, such as garlic extract, may help extend the Hayflick Limit.

DNA DAMAGE/REPAIR

DNA (**deoxyribonucleic acid**) is the molecule from which all life flows. It holds the blueprint of an organism encoded in genes. DNA is the indispensable part of the cell. Other structures, such as RNA, tions in the genes. On the other hand, when DNA is lost or damaged beyond repair, it cannot be replaced.

DNA damage can result in two principal outcomes: (1) the cell dies or (2) the cell mutates, which means that one or more of its genes lose or change their properties. The vast majority of mutations are either neutral or harmful. A small number of mutations, provided they occur in the germ cells (the cells that generate sperm or oocytes), may provide survival traits.

Substances that can damage DNA and cause mutations are called **mutagens**. Free radicals are the most common mutagens; other examples are N-nitroso compounds, aldehydes, asbestos and coal tar. Most mutagens are also carcinogens (cancer-causing substances).

DNA is constantly bombarded by mutagens. Most mutagens, like oxygen free radicals or some aldehydes are normal by-products of metabolism and cannot be avoided. However others, like environmental pollutants can be avoided, but with considerable effort and expense. Still others, like cigarette smoke or acetaldehyde (a product of alcohol breakdown in the body), are caused by our own bad habits. Different types of radiation also cause mutations; the damage produced by UV-radiation is limited mainly to the skin, cornea and retina, while high-energy radiation such as X-rays can cause mutations anywhere in the body.

The idea that the accumulation of mutations may be an important mechanism in the aging process is by no means new. Many studies have shown that species with better DNA repair mechanisms suffer fewer mutations and have a longer life span. Humans have the longest life span and the best repair system among mammals.

The frequency of mutations increases with age. One probable reason is that as we age, mutations cripple repair mechanisms, allowing more and more mutations and DNA lesions to accumulate. Also, our bodies generate more free radicals as we age, and as a consequence, more mutations and other DNA lesions. In fact, the free radical theory and the DNA damage/repair theory of aging are close cousins because DNA is one of the primary "victims" of free radicals.

DNA damage can be reduced. The first step is to limit environmental damage, like cigarette smoking and overexposure to the sun. While it is said that quitting smoking is harder than giving up heroin, at the very least, some of the effects of smoking can be reduced by switching to low tar brands. If you wish to spend time in the sun, apply sunscreen with SPF 15 or greater, with both UVA and UVB-blocking ingredients. Due to the optics of the earth's atmosphere, the morning and late afternoon sun has fewer UV-rays, so these are the ideal times for tanning. Another step you can take to reduce DNA damage is to keep your antioxidant defenses in good working order by eating plenty of fruits and vegetables and take antioxidant supplements.

At present, there is no easy way to improve the efficiency of cellular DNA repair. These complex substances involve many different enzymes. In each species, the DNA repair system has a specific standard of quality and it has a certain margin of error. Incorrect or incomplete repairs lead to mutations, the driving force behind genetic change and evolutionary change. An increase in the rate of mutations causes the species to evolve faster, but also shortens the life span of the individual organism. The reverse is also true. That is why an organism with a perfect repair system is extremely unlikely to appear

organism with a perfect repair system is extremely unlikely to appear in the natural course of our species evolution.

Humans have a more effective DNA repair system than most species: giving us the ability to age at a slower rate. Paradoxically, our fairly efficient repair system is an obstacle to evolving into a longer lived species. In our view, humans are far more likely to improve their DNA repair through science than through evolution.

GLYCATION AND CROSS-LINKING

Free radicals are a potential cause of random damage to vital body systems. Many reactive chemicals can do the same. Acetaldehyde, formed in the liver after ingesting alcohol, can damage almost any cellular structure. So can many substances in cigarette smoke or even in overfried foods. Of course, man does not live by bread alone, but avoiding alcohol, smoking or limiting fatty foods can help. However, there is one potentially damaging substance that we cannot live without - glucose.

Glucose is the most common carbohydrate found in food. It is the main structural unit of starch and a component of sucrose (table sugar), providing most energy derived from bread, cereals, pasta, and many other foods. The level of glucose in the blood is one of the most important physiological parameters. Glucose is the primary fuel of the brain, and if the level of glucose drops below a certain level for a long enough period of time a person will lose consciousness, lapse into a coma and die. High blood glucose seen in diabetes is also harmful, although the immediate consequences are less dramatic. To avoid dangerous swings in glucose levels, the body has a sophisticated system for maintaining levels within an appropriate range. Some reserve glucose is always stored in the liver in the form of glycogen, a polymer similar to starch. In addition, the liver can synthesize glucose from protein if needed. During starvation, the body breaks down muscle protein to provide the central nervous system with glucose.

Thus, the body ensures that glucose is always present in our blood. But glucose is actually a double-edged sword. In addition to its role as a vital cellular fuel, glucose is a substance that can cause damage by reacting randomly with proteins and DNA. This process is called **glycation** or **Maillard reaction**. A common example of Maillard reaction is the browning and hardening of pie crust. A somewhat similar process occurs in the body with a number of negative consequences. In particular, glycated enzymes often fail to work as well as they should. Protein glycation is believed to be one of the primary causes of cataracts, reducing the solubility of lens proteins, making them precipitate, leading to the loss of transparency.

Perhaps the worst consequence of glycation is cross-linking, which is the formation of chemical bridges between proteins or other large molecules. A material that undergoes cross-linking becomes harder, less elastic and tends to tear or crack. Cross-linking is responsible for the hardening of a rubber mat or a garden hose left in the sun. In the body, cross-linking causes hardening of arteries, wrinkling of the skin, and stiffening of joints.

An extreme example of the damage caused by glycation and cross-linking is found in diabetes. Diabetics have abnormally high rates of glycation and cross-linking as a result of elevated blood glucose which, over time, leads to severe damage to blood vessels, nerves, kidneys and other tissue.

Glucose is only one of the major cross-linkers. Cigarette smoke, UV radiation, heavy metals (such as mercury or lead), peroxides and aldehydes are all potent cross-linkers. Free radicals promote and accelerate essentially all types of cross-linking and are also cross-linkers themselves. Different types of tissue suffer from different types of cross-linking. Most of the cross-linking in the skin is usually a result of exposure to the sun; cross-linking in the lungs is due to reactive substances in tobacco tar, while glycation and free radicals are largely responsible for cross-linking in the kidneys and arterial walls.

There are a number of things you can do to reduce or even reverse cross-linking. Minimizing sun exposure or using sun block can reduce cross-linking in the skin; limiting alcohol consumption reduces the formation of acetaldehyde in the liver. Supplemental and dietary antioxidants that are free radical scavengers, reduce the rate of most types of cross-linking.

Maintaining optimal glucose tolerance is critical to minimizing glycation and cross-linking. As aging is generally accompanied by a decline in glucose tolerance higher levels of blood glucose are produced. Many factors contribute to this decline including stress and possibly, our central aging clock. You can find out how well your body tolerates glucose by asking your doctor for a glucose tolerance test. You can also improve your body's tolerance to glucose by exercising, eating a high fiber diet low in saturated fats and avoiding stress. Some nutritional supplements may also be helpful: chromium picolinate improves glucose tolerance in individuals with overt or marginal chromium deficiency, lipoic acid, coenzyme Q10, and various adaptogens like Siberian Ginseng, also help normalize blood glucose. Some nutrients that improve the sensitivity of the hypothalmus to negative feedback appear to improve glucose tolerance as well. A perfect example is melatonin.

Unlike mutations which tend to be permanent, cross-linking can be partially reversed because cells are able to manufacture replacement units for many cellular structures.

With the onset of age, the process of cross-linking begins to outpace the process of repair. If, however, the rate of cross-linking is reduced, the body can slowly replace damaged and dysfunctional structures, reversing some of the signs of aging. Even skin wrinkles can show visible improvement. Unfortunately, the rate of replacement of cross-linked parts is slow; improvement takes months and in some cases, years.

Protease, an enzyme that digests protein, may help to increase the elimination rate of cross-linked molecular debris. These enzymes can break up large cross-linked aggregates of collagen and other proteins into smaller pieces that are easier for the body to eliminate. Some proteases are found in food; the best known being bromelain in raw pineapples and papain in papaya. These enzymes are also available as supplements from any well-stocked health food store. Proteases can be used as a digestive aid, especially beneficial in the elderly who often can't produce enough of their own digestive enzymes. On the other hand, significant amounts of these enzymes find their way into the bloodstream and can remove cross-linked molecules in tissue. Bromelain was found to be especially effective. To increase its absorption into the bloodstream, it should be taken between meals.

Proteases, however, should be used with extreme caution, especially if taken on an empty stomach. They can irritate gastrointestinal lesions (ulcers, gastritis or canker sores). Papain is used in some skin rejuvenation preparations to break cross-linked collagen and promote gentle peeling.

Accumulation of Waste

In a country like the U.S., we throw out to approximately 10 pounds of garbage per day. If we multiply this by our population, we get around a trillion pounds of garbage a year. In our society, waste often exceeds production.

Some experts believe this problem will lead to catastrophic changes in our climate, coastlines and agricultural production. Environmental projections show that if the current problem continues, it will eventually lead to catastrophe.

It is amazing how many similarities there are between the environmental predicament facing mankind, and the aging process facing the human body.

Our metabolism constantly produces waste. Most of it is eliminated through breathing, urine, feces and perspiration. The easiest wastes to eliminate are small soluble molecules like urea, electrolytes and carbon dioxide. Larger molecules, such as proteins or nucleic acids, must be broken down before they can be excreted or used by the body as fuel. Cells have special digestive enzymes that break down unwanted or damaged proteins and nucleic acids into removable or usable units. Especially hard to eliminate is waste that results from random cross-linking and other unplanned reactions between cellular structures; particularly proteins. These molecular aggregates are usually large, poorly soluble and difficult to break down. Most damaged or cross-linked proteins are chopped up by intracellular proteases (protein-digesting enzymes) and become large unmanageable clumps. Evidence indicates that low cellular protease activity favor the formation of a large aggregate of molecular waste. For digesting large chunks of tough waste, cells have special **organelles** called **lysosomes** that are essentially membrane sacs filled with a variety of concentrated, aggressive digestive enzymes.

Despite the body's garbage disposal system, some types of waste accumulate over time. When neurons from the brains of young and old animals are seen under the microscope, there are some remarkable differences: the cytoplasm of old neurons contain strange yellowish deposits not found in young neurons. These are deposits of lipofuscin, an age pigment invariably found in the tissues of old animals and humans. Age pigments are a group of substances which accumulate in various aging tissues, and appear to have no useful function. Most age pigments are poorly degradable, insoluble by-products of various physiological and pathological processes. They are not chemically aggressive, but take up progressively more space and eventually begin to interfere with normal cellular functions.

Lipofuscin is the most prevalent and best studied of the aging pigments. It invariably accumulates in most tissues, especially in heart muscle, skeletal muscle and the brain. For quite some time, it had been considered a relatively innocuous by-product of normal aging and some disease states. There is now much evidence that lipofuscin is a significant contributor to aging and age-related diseases.

The accumulation of lipofuscin is closely related to other mechanisms of aging: free radicals and cross-linking. It was found that lipofuscin is an end result of free radical damage. *Lipids* (fat like compounds that are an essential part of cell membranes) are very easily damaged by oxygen free radicals, a process called lipid peroxidation. Lipid peroxides react with other lipids and proteins eventually forming large insoluble clusters. Cells try to break down such clusters with proteases and lysosomes, but are not always successfully. Aggregates of cross-linked molecular garbage that can not be digested eventually turn into lipofuscin deposits. It would appear that the greatest accumulation of lipofuscin occurs in cells that burn large amounts of fuel and rarely or never divide. Understandably, the more fuel that is consumed, the more free radicals are generated and the more cross-linked garbage is formed. It is not quite clear why frequently dividing cells do not accumulate much lipofuscin. One possible explanation is a greater activity of proteases and lysosomes in such cells.

Not all cells divide. Three main categories of cells that do not are neurons (brain cells), heart muscle cells and skeletal muscle cells. Accumulation of lipofuscin appears to contribute to age-related impairment in these tissues. All cellular processes are dependent on a normal flow of nutrients and other molecules within cells. Lipofuscin may damage tissue by mechanically obstructing normal flow, reducing the delivery of fuel and slowing down the elimination of wastes. The amount of lipofuscin in cells may exceed half of the cell's volume which is more than enough to disrupt normal traffic of molecules.

There is a correlation between the severity of dementia and congestive heart failure and the corresponding amount of lipofuscin in neurons and heart muscle cells correspondingly.

Many things affect the accumulation rate of lipofuscin. Any process that promotes free radical formation or impairs the body's antioxidant defenses promotes the growth of lipofuscin deposits. The most common of these factors is stress. Stress raises metabolic rates in the nervous system, heart muscles and skeletal tissue, causing more free radicals to be generated. There is also overwhelming evidence that stress increases lipid peroxidation, the first step in lipofuscin formation. When rats were subjected to 24 or 48 hour immobilization stress, the amount of lipofuscin in their neurons increased by 29% and 38% respectively. Another important factor in the rate of lipofuscin accumulation is the activity of cellular proteases. Young rats who received protease inhibitors (drugs that reduce protease activity) had a dramatic increase in lipofuscin deposits.

Ceroid, another aging pigment, in many ways resembles lipofuscin.

Ceroid is also an end-result of lipid peroxidation and appears to be closely related to vitamin E deficiency. An overt vitamin E deficiency is uncommon. Some gastrointestinal and liver diseases that impair the absorption of fat and fat-soluble vitamins may cause vitamin E deficiency and ceroid accumulation. Another possible cause of marginal vitamin E deficiency is a diet containing large amounts of fried foods or unsaturated fat. The principal type of fat in vegetable oil is easily oxidized and can quickly destroy vitamin E, but uncooked vegetable oil contains appreciable amounts of vitamin E - enough to offset any losses associated with high consumption of unsaturated fat. Frying and other forms of cooking deplete vitamin E from vegetable oils. High consumption of cooked, unsaturated fat may not only accelerate ceroid accumulation, but also may depress the immune system and promote some types of cancer. If your diet includes many fried foods or contains cooked unsaturated fat (e.g. French fries), a good vitamin E supplement can redress the balance.

Another pigment, **amyloid**, is sometimes found in various tissues of apparently healthy older people. More often, however, amyloid accumulation is associated with chronic infections or inflammatory diseases. The mechanism of amyloid accumulation is still somewhat mysterious. Amyloid deposits contain immunoglobulins (proteins involved in the immune response) cross-linked with other proteins, which suggests a possible autoimmune attack. The incidence of autoimmune conditions increase with age which may contribute to the accumulation of amyloid in some of the elderly. Large amyloid deposits may cause life-threatening conditions, such as heart or kidney failure.

It may be possible to slow down or even reverse the accumulation of age pigments. The first step is to improve antioxidant defenses and reduce exposure and vulnerability to stress. Due to their ability to block lipid peroxidation lipid soluble antioxidants, such as vitamin E and lipoic acid, are especially important in slowing down the accumulation of lipofuscin and ceroid. Improving glucose tolerance should reduce the rate of cross-linking reactions in neurons, and therefore slow down the growth of age pigment deposits. Several neuroactive drugs and nutrients were shown to reduce deposits of lipofuscin and ceroid in the brain. In particular, meclofenoxate and Deanol (dimethylaminoethanol p-acetamidobenzoate) were shown to reduce lipofuscin deposits in neurons in several animal species, including rodents, pigs and monkeys. It appears that the activity of both these drugs is due to dimethylaminoethanol (DMAE) which is a part of their structure. DMAE is a nutrient found in small quantities in fish and other foods, and available over-the-counter in health food stores. Like these drugs, DMAE was shown to improve various cognitive activities, such as memory, concentration and learning. In some studies, DMAE was found to increase the life span of rodents. It is still unclear how neuroactive substances shrink the deposits of age pigments in neurons. One possibility is that they activate proteases and lysosomes, and increase the amount of intracellular water, which lead to accelerated waste disposal.

CHAPTER 3

ADDING YEARS TO YOUR LIFE. ADDING LIFE TO YOUR YEARS.

What if it were possible to add another twenty years to your life - years filled with disease, suffering and infirmities. Would you still consider it worthwhile?

Chances are the answer would be no. After all, what's the point of extending one's life without improving its quality? People often joke about dying: "live fast, die young and have a good looking corpse." However macabre, many would find this alternative a lot less bleak, humiliating and frustrating than living to an old age wearing a pair of diapers.

Indeed, "old age" to many of us is synonymous with "chronic disease." Certainly, there are a group of diseases called **degenerative** or **age-related diseases** whose frequency dramatically increases with age. In technologically advanced countries these diseases account for approximately 80% of all deaths. Preventing or delaying these diseases can not only increase life expectancy, but make those added years more healthy, more productive and enjoyable.

The term **degenerative disease** implies conditions not caused by an infection, injury or hardship, but by some common slowly acting force related to lifestyle. These diseases include **atherosclerosis**, the main cause of heart disease and stroke, cancer, hypertension, noninsulin-dependent diabetes the type of diabetes that usually develops after forty, **Alzheimer's disease** the most common cause of senile dementia, **osteoporosis** brittle bones, arthritis and prostate enlargement. Age-related decline in the immune system, although not a dis

CAUSES OF DEATH
Heart disease*
Cancer*
Stroke*
Accidents
Chronic obstructive Lung disease
Pneumonia and Influenza**
Diabetes mellitus***
Suicide
Chronic liver diseases and Cirrhosis
Homicide

* Age-related diseases
** Most cases are precipitated by age-related decline in the immune function
*** Diabetes type II (noninsulin-dependent) is age-related and accounts for over 90 % of all cases.

Table2. The ten leading causes of death in the US Source National Center for Health Statistics, Annual Summary of Births, Marriages Divorces, and Deaths, 1990.

ease by itself, is largely responsible for the deaths from pneumonia and influenza that are quite common among the elderly.

Degenerative diseases are often looked upon as a curse of modern times. Many people believe that they are the direct and inevitable outcome of the so-called "civilized world."

Today heart disease, stroke and cancer are directly linked to the cause of two-thirds of all deaths in our culture. Of course, lifestyle plays an important role in the development of these and other age related diseases. But equally important, we live longer than previous generations, giving us more time to develop degenerative diseases and as a result, more time to treat them.

When prehistoric man roamed the earth, sheer survival made excellent health a necessity. Early man had to be in great shape to battle carnivores with nothing more than a spear. Something as trivial as a common cold or a lack of plumbing often posed a mortal threat to our ancestors. Even a slight decline in stress resistance or immunity could have led many a man to an early exit. Next, there were no antibiotics, intensive care units or even sanitized rest rooms.

The relative safety of modern society enables us to survive for a longer period of time with relatively low stress resistance and a sluggish immune system. It seems as though we live just long enough to develop degenerative diseases. Animals living in captivity have a much longer life span than those raised in the wild. Yet captive animals tend to develop degenerative diseases: ironically, the very same diseases found in man - atherosclerosis, diabetes and cancer, etc.

The total number of degenerative diseases rises well into the hundreds, yet surprisingly, few of them account for the vast majority of deaths. Why is that so? Why are degenerative diseases synonymous with aging? The answer lies in the similarity between the mechanisms of aging and the causes of degenerative diseases.

In other words, the same process that leads to aging also contributes to degenerative diseases.

(1) **Free radicals** contribute to most degenerative diseases, including atherosclerosis, cancer, dementia, cataracts and arthritis. They do so through a variety of mechanisms. One of the best known examples is the oxidation of **LDL** (low density lipoproteins). LDL are fatty globules in the blood whose function is to deliver cholesterol to the tissues. When LDL are oxidized they become "sticky" and adhere to arterial plaques causing them to flourish. Eventually, the plaque blocks the flow of blood to vital organs. Free radicals promote LDL oxidation while certain antioxidants, such as vitamin E or lipoic acid inhibit their activity. Several studies have demonstrated that high doses of vitamin E (400 - 1200 I.U. per day) reduce the risk of heart disease, presumably blocking free radicals and preventing LDL oxidation.

(2) **The central aging clock** located in the brain is another driving force behind degenerative disease causes a variety of gradual hormonal and metabolic shifts that favor the onset of disease. For instance, insulin excess and decreased glucose tolerances increase the risks of atherosclerosis, hypertension, diabetes and obesity. Also excessive secretion of steroid hormones in response to stress contributes to the

development of atherosclerosis, diabetes, obesity, age-related diseases, impaired immunity and cancer. High prolactin levels are a factor in prostate enlargement.

(3) **Glycation and cross-linking** harden arteries and make them more fragile, increasing the risk of hypertension, atherosclerosis and stroke; these processes also promote cataracts and immune dysfunction.

(4) **Age pigments**, such as lipofuscin and ceroid, which are a result of free radical damage and cross-linking, contribute to dementia and heart failure.

(5) **The role of the cellular aging clock** (the Hayflick Limit) in degenerative disease is less easily understood. On one hand, the Hayflick Limit may represent an important mechanism in preventing unlimited cell growth - some scientists believing that it has evolved as an anticancer security system. It may also contribute to the decline in the functional and regenerative capacity of tissues with high cell division rates. An example is that a decreased ability of the cells in blood vessels linings to divide, may contribute to the development of arterial plaque.

(6) Finally, an important factor in both aging and degenerative diseases is **stress**. As we've described, stress accelerates all aspects of the aging process and also increases the risk of degenerative diseases. Some diseases are more likely to be precipitated by stress than others. For example, hypertension can be dramatically worsened by stress. Perhaps it is because stress causes increased heart rate, constriction of blood vessels and reduction of body fluids. Intense stress may escalate with glucose intolerance to diabetes, throwing the diabetic into a life-threatening situation. Hormonal and metabolic changes caused by stress also contribute to atherosclerosis, immune dysfunction and an increased risk of cancer.

Reducing stress or improving stress resistance is vital not only for life extension, but also self-preservation. **Adaptogens** (the substances that mitigate and optimize the stress response) were found beneficial in preventing or even reversing many degenerative diseases.

Another important factor in degenerative diseases is that they rarely appear alone. A person is either free of degenerative diseases or suffers from several at once. Some of the combinations frequently found together are atherosclerosis, hypertension and obesity or, atherosclerosis, hypertension, arthritis and prostate enlargement. One possible explanation for this clustering is that many degenerative diseases are caused by the same or similar mechanisms as aging itself.

Some gereontologists believe that degenerative diseases are simply an expected normal by-product of aging, and can be used as markers of biological vs. chronological age. However, there is quite a lot more to it. Most degenerative diseases have multiple causes and contributing factors. Some of these are related to the mechanisms of aging while others are not. For instance, a deficiency in folic acid contributes to atherosclerosis and heart diseases (by increasing the blood levels of homocysteine, an atherosclerosis-promoting metabolite), but has little to do with the aging process itself. On the other hand, another factor in atherosclerosis, lipid peroxidation, is a result of free radical damage, an important aging mechanism.

Insulin excesses, a common endocrine abnormality of aging caused by age-related decreases in carbohydrate tolerance, is an important contributor to the development of several degenerative diseases and abnormalities, including hypertension, atherosclerosis, obesity, diabetes, possibly depressed immunity and even increased risk of cancer. This cluster of disorders often seen in people with insulin excess has received the chilling name, "Syndrome X" in medical literature. The causes of age-related insulin excess are still somewhat unclear, but appear to be a part of endocrine shifts driven by the central aging clock.

To make matters even more confusing, degenerative diseases themselves tend to accelerate many of the mechanisms of aging. Diabetes is probably the most dramatic example. It intensifies free radical formation, glycation and crosslinking and also appears to speed up the central aging clock. Another example is atherosclerosis, which reduces blood supply to the tissues by clogging arteries. When blood flow is too low, the cellular antioxidant systems lose their efficiency., even though there is still enough oxygen to generate free radicals; the consequence of this is more free radical damage and faster aging.

The bottom line is that life extension and disease prevention are not two distinct undertakings - both fit into one comprehensive strategy because the mechanisms that cause aging and degenerative diseases are largely one and the same. In addition to extending life span, blocking the mechanisms of aging has the more immediate benefit of preventing degenerative diseases.

CHAPTER 4

AGING AND HORMONES: A TWO WAY STREET

ENDOCRINE SYSTEM AND HORMONES

Few things in the universe, if any, are more complex than the human body. The sum total of cells alone is well into the tens of trillions. Literally, each of them is a world unto itself. If each cell were the size of a bee, the hive would dwarf the Pyramids.

How is it then that all these cells manage to work together so flawlessly? In a beehive, coordination of effort is achieved through efficient communication between different types of bees. The bees release special chemicals called pheromones that travel through the air and induce other bees to perform specific actions needed for the common good. This is somewhat similar to the communication system between cells in the human body. They can "talk" to each other through chemical messages carried via the bloodstream.

The **endocrine system** is the primary system responsible for the efficient coordination of body functions. It consists of three parts; the hypothalamus, the pituitary, and the peripheral endocrine glands. To perform its duties, the endocrine system uses **hormones**, which are special messenger molecules, transmitting instructions from the endocrine system to all other organs in the body, as well as between different levels of the endocrine system itself. When a hormone reaches its target cell, it interacts with a receptor, something of a molecular "push-button" for eliciting a specific response. For each hormone there are one or more types of receptors that respond to it.

Each cell's response to hormones is dependent upon what types of receptors it has.

Like a beehive, the endocrine system has a chain of command. The hypothalamus is a small structure at the base of the brain that serves as the strategic command center for the endocrine system. The hypothalamus processes the information about the outside world by analyzing the signals sent to it by the nervous system, and monitors the body's internal environment by analyzing blood composition. If the hypothalamus "decides" that some physiological changes are to be made, it sends an order to the pituitary, the master gland of the endocrine system. You can say that if the hypothalamus were the board of directors, the pituitary would be the CEO.

The pituitary gland is located in the exact center of the brain, just beneath the hypothalamus and has two main lobes, the anterior and posterior. The pituitary is capable of secreting more than a dozen different hormones required for the regulation of the body's metabolism, growth, reproduction and stress responses.

When the hypothalamus has "decided" what changes to make, it secretes special hormones called **releasing hormones**. Depending on the releasing hormone sent, the pituitary secretes a corresponding hormone into the bloodstream. Most hormones released by the pituitary act on peripheral endocrine glands, such as the thyroid, adrenal, and sex glands. Peripheral endocrine glands function as middle management, in turn, releasing hormones of their own which act on specific organs or tissues making them perform specific tasks.

A good way of showing how the endocrine system works is to look at what it does when the body is under stress, like giving a speech. As the hypothalamus "senses" the stressful situation, it releases corticotropin-releasing hormone (CRH) which causes the pituitary to release another hormone called adrenocorticotropic hormone (aka ACTH, or corticotropin). ACTH acts on the adrenal glands (small glands located just above the kidneys) which causes them to release stress steroids that act on various organs and tissues. This chain of events is responsible for unleashing the many physiological changes seen during any stressful situation including the elevation of blood glucose, the increased breakdown of lean tissue and the suppression of the immune system.

The underlying principle of the endocrine system is something called **negative feedback**. After the hypothalamus has sent a signal down the line to set in motion certain changes in the body, there is a feedback signal from the periphery to ensure that the system's response is not excessive. In other words, it protects the system from overtaxing itself. The hormones secreted by the pituitary and peripheral endocrine glands serve as a means for providing this feedback. If the hypothalamus senses that the level of a certain hormone is too high, it discontinues the initial order. This prevents excessive swings in hormone levels and helps maintain the body's hormonal balance. Before we go any further, let's get back to the subject of stress hormones. When the hypothalamus senses too high a level of ACTH or stress steroids it stops releasing CRH. This creates feedback loops that limit the stress response which if unchecked, can prove devastating.

HOW AGING AFFECTS THE ENDOCRINE SYSTEM AND VICE VERSA

As we age, the endocrine system undergoes profound changes. The levels of many hormones decline while others are produced in great excess.

Sluggishness and slow metabolism in the elderly are partly due to the decline in levels of thyroid hormones; and a decreased sex drive may result from low levels of sex hormones, particularly testosterone.

Until recently, it was generally thought that age-related changes in key hormone levels were an inevitable consequence of aging, and should not be tampered with. Replacement of deficient hormones was viewed as "giving a unicycle to a quadriplegic." However, there is one important exception: estrogen replacement therapy in postmenopausal women. This practice has become part of standard care for postmenopausal women over the past four decades. Many studies have

HORMONE	CHANGE WITH AGE	POSSIBLE CONSEQUENCES
Growth hormone	↓	Loss of lean body mass; decreased immunity; decreased stress resistance; lower metabolic rate; abdominal obesity; depression; decreased sex drive
Thyroid hormones	↓	Decreased metabolic rate; weight gain; lassitude
Insulin (in nondiabetics)	↑	Atherosclerosis; hypertension; abdominal obesity
Insulin (in type II diabetics)	↑ or ↓	High blood sugar leading to atherosclerosis; small vessel damage; kidney, nerve, eye damage.
Cortisol	↑	Loss of lean body; depressed immunity; insulin resistance; elevated blood sugar, cholesterol, and free fatty acids; progression of atherosclerosis and hypertension; abdominal obesity
DHEA	↕	Loss of lean body mass and increase in body fat; low stress resistance; depression or lack of well-being; decreased sex drive; dry skin; decline in some aspects of immunity
Testosterone(men)	↕	Decreased libido; loss of muscle mass
Dehydrotestosterone (in men)	↕	Prostate enlargement; male pattern
Estrogens (in postmenopausal women)	↕	Increased risk of heart diseases and stroke (due to atherosclerosis); osteoporosis; vaginal dryness
Melatonin	↕	Decreased immunity; insomnia or lack of restful sleep; increased risk of cancer
Gonadotropins (FSH, LH)	↕	Hot flashes (usually in women)
Prolactin (in men)	↓	Prostate enlargement; impotence; impaired function of the testes

Table 3. Factors believed to speed up or slow down the central aging clock located in the hypothalamus and related brain structures.

demonstrated the benefits of estrogen replacement, including lower risk of osteoporosis, heart disease and stroke. Estrogen replacement tends to cause a modest increase in the rate of breast cancer, but this is partially offset by a decline in other forms of cancer.

The more we know about the aging process, the clearer it becomes that age-related hormonal changes are not just a side effect of aging, but also one of its causes. Many debilitating manifestations of aging appear to be linked to low levels of growth hormone, DHEA, melatonin, thyroid hormones, testosterone and estrogen. The restoration of youthful levels of these hormones were shown to help retard or partly reverse the aging process.

There are many contributing factors to age-related hormonal imbalances, but the main cause appears to be the **central aging clock** located in the hypothalamus and adjacent brain structures.

As we age, the efficiency of the feedback loops between the hypothalamus and other endocrine glands decline, causing the body's internal environment to gradually deviate from its optimal state.

Homeostasis is like the thermostat in your home. When the temperature drops, the thermostat's sensor detects changes and turns on the heater. When the house becomes too warm, the thermostat shuts off the heater.

In a young body, all thermostats are extremely sensitive to temperature changes and do not allow the "house" to overheat or cool down too much. With age, the thermostat becomes less sensitive and we begin to see a lot of deviations from so-called normal physiology.

In the body, the main sensors that monitor the internal environment are located in the hypothalamus. According to Dilman's theory of the central aging clock, these sensors lose their acuity with age which impair the efficiency of feedback loops. This results in disturbances in homeostasis and undesirable changes in body chemistry.

Dilman reasoned that, in order to develop, the body must shift its homestasis through the process of gradually blunting the hypothalamic sensors. This is precisely what the central aging clock does. In fact, it should actually be called a growth and development clock because it paces growth and development of the body. The problem is that after age twenty to twenty-five this clock continues ticking, but at that point the result is not growth and maturation. It is just the opposite: accelerated aging, increased risk of degenerative-diseases, and the impaired ability to adapt to stress.

What does all this have to do with age-related changes in the levels of various hormones? Apparently, quite a lot. These hormonal changes are the main tool by which the hypothalamus implements a program of development and then a program of aging. But the hypothalmus cannot do it on its own. It's function is that of a policy maker, not an executive. To implement this "strategic policy, " the hypothalamus gives orders to the pituitary gland which releases a host of hormones. Some pituitary hormones act on other endocrine glands making them release hormones of their own. Still others act directly on organs and tissues. The bottom line is that the central aging clock works mainly by setting off a barrage of hormonal changes in the body. In childhood and youth these hormonal changes help the body develop. After that, however, they help push the body chemistry in the opposite direction.

What can be done to neutralize age-related hormonal changes?

One strategy is to try to slow down, or even reverse the pace of the central aging clock to remove the major cause of age-related hormonal changes. Ways to achieve this include: boosting the levels of neurotransmitters in the brain; reducing stress and optimizing the stress response; improving the ability of the tissues to respond to insulin, and reducing the levels of free radicals in the brain.

Another strategy is to replace deficient hormones. The first strategy tends to work better in younger people. In older people, a combination of the two strategies appears to provide the best results, although individual responses may vary considerably.

In the following chapters we will discuss the roles of individual hormones in the aging process and the benefits of restoring their levels to a youthful state.

CHAPTER 5

GROWTH HORMONE: THE BODY OF EVIDENCE IS GROWING

Among the "magic bullets" of life extension heralded by the press in recent years, growth hormone (GH) could arguably have the greatest impact. This remarkable hormone lives up to at least some of the hype. It is one of the key factors in stimulating growth. An underproduction of GH leads to dwarfism, and excess to gigantism or, in the case of late onset, to acromegaly, a condition characterized by the disproportionate growth of soft tissues. When the body stops growing somewhere between the ages twenty to twenty-five, GH does not lose its importance. In fact, GH helps maintain body mass and composition, facilitate healing and tissue regeneration, and stimulates the immune and other body systems. Directly or indirectly, GH affects all tissues of the body at all stages of life.

Aging is often associated with a dramatic decline in GH production. From the age twenty to sixty, the level of GH drops by about 80%. A relative GH deficiency seen in the majority of older people appears to contribute to a loss of muscle mass, slower metabolism, abdominal obesity and slow wound healing. GH is also associated with weak immunity, decreased stress resistance, loss of sex drive and other signs of aging; many of these signs appear to improve with GH replacement.

Popular interest and media coverage of GH received a boost in 1990 when Dr. Daniel Rudman and colleagues from the Medical College of Wisconsin published a study on GH replacement in the New England Journal of Medicine. The study involved 21 healthy men from sixty-one to eighty-one-years-old. Twelve men received GH injections over a period of 6 months, the other 9 men received no treatment. Those treated with GH had an average of 8.8% increase in lean body mass and a 14.4% decrease in fat; skin thickness increased by 7.1%, and density of some bones increased slightly.

Rudman's study generated a wave of overwhelming enthusiasm. However, the small size and relative lack of structure gave little credence to the study. In the past few years, several other studies of GH-replacement in older individuals were conducted, supporting some of Rudman's initial hypotheses and eliminating others. At this point, GH appears to be a valuable anti-aging tool capable of partially reversing some, but not all aspects of the aging process. Also, individuals response to GH may vary dramatically.

Growth hormone is the most abundant hormone in the human pituitary gland. It is a protein consisting of 191 amino acids. The release of GH by the pituitary is controlled mainly by chemical signals from the hypothalamus. The peak of GH production occurs in early childhood when body growth is at its peak. After puberty, the levels of GH peak and then continuously decline. After age twenty, GH levels drop at the rate of approximately 14% per decade. There is no doubt that this decline contributes throughout the aging process, although how much, is still being debated.

Why does GH production decrease with age? A definitive answer is yet to be found. What we do know is that aging does not seem to impair the capacity of the pituitary gland to release GH. One plausible hypothesis is that the central aging clock is responsible for the fall of GH levels with age. Age-related changes in the hypothalamus (the loss of sensitivity to feedback signals from the body) lead to high levels of the hormone somatostatin, which is a natural inhibitor of GH. Note: Many of the effects of GH on tissues are indirect. GH makes the liver release the hormones called somatomedins, the most important ones being IGF-1 and IGF-2, which act directly on most tissues and organs. The administration of IGF-1 to GH-deficient animals reproduces most of the effects of GH, including body size and tissue growth as well as increased protein synthesis and fat utilization. Blood levels of IGF-1 were shown to be a better indicator of the growth hormone status than the levels of GH itself. The reason for that is GH is released in bursts and remains in the bloodstream for a relatively short period of time. IGF-1, on the other hand, remains in the blood for many hours. Its levels reflect the total amount of GH released. Hence, in most clinical studies, researchers measure the levels of IGF-1 rather than GH itself.

GH ALTERS BODY COMPOSITION AND METABOLISM

The most consistent finding in GH replacement studies appears to be the change in body composition. At the age of twenty, the body consists of approximately 80% lean tissue (muscle, bone and organs) and 20% fatty or adipose tissue. As we age, the lean tissue is gradually replaced by fat at a rate of about 5% every 10 years. Physical strength, stamina, and functional capacity of many organs seem to decline in relation to the loss of lean body mass. In several studies, GH replacement was shown to reverse this process, causing lean tissue to increase and fat to decrease thereby restoring a leaner, more muscular, youthful physique. In some cases, GH replacement increased work capacity and endurance. The most dramatic change is usually seen in the loss of abdominal fat, which is a well documented risk factor for diabetes, hypertension and heart disease. In one well-designed Swedish study thirty men with abdominal obesity, forty-eight to sixty-six years old were treated with 0.0095 mg of GH per kilogram of body weight for nine months. Total body fat decreased by 9.2%, and visceral fat other than under the skin by 18.1%.

GH exerts its effects on body composition through changes in metabolism. It stimulates cells to generate more energy and synthesize more protein, prompting the growth of lean tissue. Fat stores are used up as an energy source for new tissue growth. In some studies, GH reduced cholesterol and LDL, and increased HDL levels. Several studies report the metabolic benefits of GH, including improved carbohydrate tolerance, lower blood glucose levels and increased sensitivity of tissues to insulin.

All in all, it appears that the metabolic effects of GH replacement may help slow down some of the metabolic mechanisms of aging (such as insulin resistance) and reduce the risk of cardiovascular disease.

GH AIDS IN TISSUE REGENERATION

Regeneration of atrophied or injured organs is not only necessary for health and longevity, it is also important to survival. GH seems to hold considerable promise in improving survival and accelerating recovery in some types of terrible injuries. To date, the most impressive are the results of GH therapy used in the treatment of severe burns.

A group from Harvard studied the effects of GH therapy in 54 patients with extensive burns. Half of the patients received GH. In the control group, mortality was 37%, and in the GH group 11% (about 3 1/2 times lower). Although these finding are statistically significant, larger and better-structured studies are needed to confirm this truly remarkable result. Another study conducted at the Shriner's Burn Institute found that in 40 two to eighteen-year-old patients, GH therapy reduced hospital stays from an average of 46 to 32 days (a decrease of over 30%).

Internal organs gradually atrophy with age, shrinking in size and losing functional capacity. Can growth hormone help reverse this? Based upon the scarce data available today, it might. In 1991, Dr. Rudman's study found that 12 months of GH therapy increased the liver, spleen and kidney size, as well as skin thickness and muscle mass. Even diseased organs may be able to regenerate and heal with GH therapy. In a 1996 New England Journal of Medicine study, researchers investigated the effects of GH on dilated cardiomyopathy. In this condition, the heart can not adequately adapt to the body's demand for pumping blood, resulting in the dilation of left ventricle, thinning of the heart muscle and eventually, heart failure. Three months of therapy with recombinant GH increased myocardial mass, reduced the size of the left ventricular chamber and improved circulation, myocardial function and clinical status. Several other studies on GH therapy have improved heart performance in relieving healthy elderly patients and those heart disease patients on GH therapy. Preliminary reports indicate that GH may also help in emphysema and renal failure.

GH AND IMMUNITY

It has been proven beyond any reasonable doubt that GH enhances the immune function. In fact, the decline in the levels of both GH, and melatonin could very well be responsible for much of the immune system's deterioration with age. Animals whose pituitary glands develop a severe immune deficiency is attributed mainly to the lack of GH. As we noted earlier, the most dramatic and universal age-related change in the immune system is the shrinkage of the thymus gland which serves as a "training center" for lymphocytes. Deterioration of the thymus function increases susceptibility to infection and, possibly cancer. Several studies have also demonstrated that administration of GH can help restore both the size and the function of the aged thymus.

In addition, there is evidence that GH can directly stimulate several types of the immune cells, including B- and T-lymphocytes, natural killer cells and macrophages.

GH AND DEPRESSION

There appears to be an important connection between GH levels and depression. Individuals with lower than normal levels of GH and IGF-

1 tend to have more symptoms of depression. They include a lack of energy and motivation, apathy, generally poor mood, social isolation and anxiety. In many cases, GH therapy produces a dramatic improvement in mood, energy, motivation, sex drive and overall zest for life. It remains unclear how GH accomplishes this. It may work by increasing the levels of endorphins (natural mood-elevators and painkillers) and altering the levels of various neurotransmitters to create a more youthful balance.

GH AND SEXUALITY

A genuine desire to improve sex drive and performance is often among the reasons why people embark on GH therapy. Evidence that GH can improve one's sex life is largely anecdotal. However, presently, there are no clinical studies that specifically address this issue. In a small scale study that specifically addressed this issue conducted at the University of California, researchers reported that GH therapy produced a significant increase in sexual desire among men but not women.

In their 1997 book, "Grow Young with GH," Dr. Ronald Klatz and Carol Kahn review lay surveys of GH-treated patients and opinions of clinicians experienced in GH therapy. The authors' general conclusion is that GH therapy improves at least some aspects of sexuality in the majority of patients with a few experiencing a dramatic sexual revival.

Theoretically, GH may boost sexual performance in men by improving cardiovascular function and increasing testosterone production. GH might boost libido in both men and women by raising brain levels of neurotransmitters, particularly norepinephrine, an important factor in arousal. Old age and depression often go hand in hand with decreased sexual desire. The positive effects of GH on depression may also help increase sex drive.

WHAT GH CANNOT DO

We have already learned what GH can do. Now let's take a look at what it can't do. It's definitely no cure-all or aging-stopper. As we continue to stress, the aging process is highly complex and there really are no simple answers. GH may retard or reverse some signs of aging like the loss of lean body mass and decreased immunity. However, there is a significant variation in individual responses to GH with dramatic effects in some people and minimal effects in others. People in their eighties or older appear to be less responsive to GH injections than fifty or sixty-year-olds. In one 1996 study, GH injections failed to improve some immune parameters in elderly women. In another 1996 study conducted in healthy men aged seventy or older, 6 month of therapy with physiologic doses of GH improved body composition, but failed to improve functional abilities. Frequent side effects were observed, indicating that the elderly may be more likely to be adversely effected by GH even at physiological doses. Studies in postmenopausal women indicate that GH produces only very small improvements in bone density, being far inferior in regard to estrogens.

We believe that maintaining youthful levels of growth hormone may provide life extension benefits. For most people, the safest and most affordable way to boost GH levels is through the stimulation of their own secretion (see Chapter 25 for practical details). Some individuals, carefully selected by competent physicians, may benefit from GH injections.

GROWTH HORMONE AND STRESS

The ability to overcome stress declines with age along with production of growth hormone. At this time, we cannot say with any certainty that GH deficiency contributes to the loss of stress resistance with age. However, scientists have found a number of important links between GH levels and resistance to stress.

Most importantly, GH and stress have opposite effects on lean tissue. Stress causes the breakdown of proteins for fuel and the loss of lean body mass (catabolism). Conversely, GH promotes protein synthesis and increases lean body mass (anabolism).

In a number of recent studies, scientists have attempted to counter the effects of severe stress by the administration of GH. One Spanish study investigated the ability of GH to speed up the recovery of patients from the trauma of surgery, and in particular to reduce the duration and intensity of post operative fatigue. Researchers found that low-dose GH injections (8 IU/day) minimized post-operation fatigue and prevented the loss of lean tissue which normally follows surgical stress. A New Zealand study looked at the effects of GH injections in sheep subjected to metabolic stress induced by a 70 hour fast. In fasting animals, GH treatment reduced the use of protein for fuel and partially prevented the loss of lean tissue.

What are the practical implications of the link between stress and GH? GH therapy during severe stress like surgery, trauma, burn or severe illness, may prevent some stress-related damage, including the loss of lean body mass and quite possibly the suppression of the immune function. Many studies are now in progress to evaluate this approach. In older individuals, who are less stress-resistant and tend to have diminished GH and/or IGF-1 production, the administration of GH, IGF-1 or GH-releasers during stressful situations may turn out be especially beneficial, allowing them to ride out hard times with minimal losses.

The Author's Discovery of the Anti-Aging Potential of Growth Hormone

The use of growth hormone today to delay or even reverse some signs of aging has become the darling of geriatric physicians, the media and much of the scientific community.

This supposedly "new" idea, has actually been around since the Fifties. In those days, when Dr. I. N. Todorov first suggested this approach, GH was largely considered a mystery. The entire body of knowledge on GH consisted of the fact that this hormone was known to be a key player in the growth of mammals. Nobody knew how it worked, why it worked or anything else about it, for that matter. The idea of the link between the body's GH production and aging had not even begun to emerge. As a graduate student at Kharkov State University, Ukraine, Dr. Todorov devoted his doctoral thesis to this problem. Specifically, he set out to study the effects of GH on the metabolism of nucleic acids (the key information molecules of life - DNA and RNA) in animals of different age.

The Fifties were a simpler time. Unfortunately, studying GH was not quite that simple. The first obstacle was how to obtain enough pure GH.

Today, in the era of genetic engineering, animal or human proteins can be mass-produced in the lab using designer bacteria. Getting enough GH to conduct a quantifiable study is simply a matter of placing an order with a biotech company and choosing a good overnight delivery service.

Back then, obtaining even the smallest amount of pure GH was incredibly difficult. The author had to make numerous trips to a slaughterhouse where he had to manually extract tiny pituitary glands (a sole source of GH in the body) from freshly discarded bovine heads - hundreds of them. To obtain 2-3 grams of GH required for a series of experiments, the author had to collect over a kilogram worth (about two and a half pounds) of bovine pituitary glands, each weighing 1.5-2.5 gms. Then a lengthy purification procedure was performed. Only then could the beautiful needle-like crystals of GH be obtained.

The author used this "purified biotreasure" to study biological effects of GH in the animals of different age. The study took about two years to complete and yielded very intriguing results. The older the animals, the stronger their anabolic response to repeated GH injections, i. e. the more lean tissue and vital biological molecules, such as DNA, RNA and proteins, the animals produced. The greatest effect was seen in the oldest (twenty-month-old) rats, whereas the youngest animals (one-month-old) did not respond to multiple injections at all.

These results suggested that growth hormone levels decline with age. Indeed, the levels of GH in young animals were obviously so high that the anabolic responseof tissues was already at its maximum, and additional GH had no effect. On the other hand, old animals evidently produced very little GH. So their response to GH injections was quite dramatic. In the Fifties, such a hypothesis was hard to prove because there were no accurate methods to test blood levels of GH. Later, as sophisticated measuring techniques became available, GH levels were indeed found to decline with age in all mammals.

Another important conclusion made by the author was that the ability of GH to increase the synthesis of nucleic acids and proteins (i.e. the key molecules of life) in old animals could provide a way to shift the metabolism of an old body into a younger state, and thus delay or reverse some symptoms of aging. Unfortunately, at that time, there was no way of practically testing and implementing this approach in humans. The problem lay in the species specificity of growth hormone. Bovine GH worked in rats but was ineffective in humans, presumably due to to a great difference in structure; there was no way to obtain significant quantities of human growth hormone (hGH). Only in the era of genetic engineering could this obstacle be overcome. The gene encoding hGH was isolated and inserted into bacteria with recombinant DNA techniques, creating a microscopic GH-producing machine. The resulting recombinant hGH is almost identical to its counterpart produced by the human pituitary and exerts the same biological action. In the Eighties, thirty years after the author's studies in rats, other researchers obtained similar results with hGH in humans. Today, the supply of hGH for research and therapy is virtually unlimited. Ironically, our current knowledge indicates that the injections of exogenous hGH may not be the best way to go for most people. In most cases, the best strategy is to boost one's own GH production by combining GH-releasers, diet and exercise.

CHAPTER 6

MELATONIN: SEPARATING HYPE FROM HOPE.

Over the past few years, melatonin has become one of the most widely used and misused over-the-counter supplements. According to German scientist Dr. Huether, "melatonin has made an impressive career from a stepchild of hormone research to a marketing phenomenon."

This so-called "wonder drug" owes much of its success to the miracle of modern marketing, not modern science. It is hyped by the media as a **super drug** that: slows down aging, prevents disease, cures insomnia, is nontoxic and is available on the shelf of your local drugstore at a cost of about $3 for a month's supply.

Considering all of the attention melatonin has received, people tend to view it as little more than hype. This couldn't be further from the truth. Based upon today's evidence, many experts believe that melatonin may indeed provide an impressive array of health benefits, especially in older individuals. The list of potential uses includes treatment of sleep disorders, depressed immune system, cancer, hypertension, atherosclerosis, Diabetes and Alzheimer's disease. Melatonin is a potent antioxidant that may also reduce damage caused by stress and an extensive study of melatonin in humans has just begun. At this point, most of melatonin's benefits have yet to be proven.

Although several short-term human studies are currently in the works, no long-term human studies have been completed, which leaves unclear, questions about its anti-aging potential as well as its long-term side effects. Mice who received melatonin throughout the second half of their lives had a 20% increase in life span. When it comes to humans, it may be a long time before we have any definitive answers on melatonin's effects on human life span.

Before we go any further, let's begin at the beginning. Melatonin is a molecule found in every plant and animal on earth. After emerging as part of a living organism about three billion years ago, its essential structure remains unchanged. This type of structural conservatism is usually found only in unchanged essential substances of life.

When melatonin was first discovered in the late Fifties by Yale dermatologist, Dr. Aaron Lerner, scientists had no idea of its capabilities. For almost 2 decades, its only known function was to regulate sleep and hibernation. As research methods improved, melatonin was shown to affect many body systems, especially the nervous and immune system, and possibly the central aging clock.

Melatonin production peaks before puberty and drops precipitously. In fact, recent research indicates that the decrease in melatonin during the early teens is one of the key factors in the onset of sexual maturation. It was found that children whose puberty was delayed tend to have excessively high melatonin levels and those who mature unusually early often produce too little melatonin. After maturity, the levels of melatonin continue to drop. In forty year-olds, melatonin levels are usually about 1/3 of those found in young adults. Melatonin is barely detectable in sixty-year-olds. This decline appears to be not just a consequence of aging, but actually a contributing factor to the aging process.

As we mentioned, food restriction is the most potent known method of increasing life expectancy in animals. Researchers found that food restriction causes a marked rise in melatonin levels, and may be one of the mechanisms through which restricting food intake increases life span. A definitive answer, however, can be obtained only by a study in which animals are put on a restricted diet in addition to being treated with a drug that suppresses melatonin production. If they fail to live longer than control animals, then we can presume that melatonin is essential for some of the anti-aging effects of food restriction.

The ability of melatonin to affect the rate of sexual development and extend life in animals may have to do with the central aging clock. This clock paces both the development and aging of the body. Melatonin appears to affect the central aging clock by altering the way the hypothalamus communicates with other organs. In particular, it makes the hypothalamus more responsive to the feedback from other parts of the body.

Like any large organization whose management fails to respond to feedback from employees or customers, our bodies too will eventually deteriorate and fail if the lines of communication are broken. Melatonin may actually help to slow this breakdown.

MELATONIN IS A POTENT ANTIOXIDANT

Melatonin is a very versatile molecule, capable of doing many jobs simultaneously. Among other things, it is a potent antioxidant. Most antioxidants are either water or fat-soluble and therefore, can protect only the "watery"or "fatty" areas of the cell. For instance, vitamin E is very effective in protecting cellular membranes, which are "fatty," but cannot protect DNA and most proteins. Conversely, glutathione, a key water-soluble antioxidant, protects DNA and proteins but not the membranes. Melatonin, on the other hand, protects all parts of the cell's structure and is several times more effective than either vitamin E or glutathione.

Some antioxidants, such as vitamin C and beta-carotene, can under certain circumstances, do the opposite of what they normally do. Instead of capturing free radicals, these antioxidants may start to produce them. For instance, vitamin C can generate free radicals in the presence of free iron occurring with an injury or an infection. Melatonin has never even shown the slightest hint of being this kind of troublemaker.

From the standpoint of life extension, protecting DNA is the most important of all its antioxidant activities. Damaged membranes can be repaired and damaged proteins can be replaced. But some of the free radical damage to DNA is completely irreversible. As you may remember from high school biology, DNA is the very foundation of life itself; it holds the genetic blueprints to any organism in the cell. With these blueprints you can repair almost anything, given enough time and energy. Trouble starts when this blueprint is damaged. Melatonin was found to be remarkably effective in protecting DNA. In some animal studies, melatonin reduced free radical damage to DNA caused by toxic chemicals by as much as 99%. Further, melatonin seems to have the ability to accumulate in the cell's nucleus so that its concentration near DNA is higher than in the rest of the body. This makes melatonin, DNA's "personal bodyguard."

As an antioxidant, melatonin has yet another remarkable attribute. It stimulates the production of glutathione peroxidase, one of the key free-radical scavenging enzymes. Generally, adding antioxidants to cells reduces the production of free radical scavenging enzymes. It is as if the cell were thinking "Why should I use my own antioxidants when I can get them free without using up any energy?" As a result, many antioxidant supplements produce little overall improvement in antioxidant protection. Melatonin is unique in that it both provides direct antioxidant shielding and stimulates the cell's internal free radical scavenging systems.

MELATONIN AND THE BRAIN

Melatonin affects the brain in a number of ways. The pineal gland, the center of melatonin production, is located at the very center of the brain. When produced, melatonin is quickly distributed throughout the brain and readily absorbed by neurons.

One of the first discovered functions of melatonin was its role in regulating the sleep/wake cycle. At night, the levels of melatonin are several times higher than during the day which serves to promote general relaxation and induce restful sleep. The incidence of insomnia and poor quality of sleep in the elderly is partly due to insufficient melatonin production.

Today, millions of people use a melatonin supplement as a sleep aid. Unlike common sleep-inducing drugs, melatonin usually produces no adverse side effects and does not disturb the normal structure of sleep (normal sleep consists of several phases comprising a particular pattern critical for optimal health).

Melatonin is also commonly taken to reduce the effects of jet lag or shift-work. If you take melatonin at the time when it isn't normally produced by your body, you will fool it into "thinking" that your body should start its nightly cycle: relax, reduce heart rate and general activity and go to sleep. After several days of such off-phase melatonin supplementation, you will have shifted you sleep/wake cycle by the required number of hours.

There is some preliminary evidence that melatonin is a very effective protector of the brain against free radicals. As the brain consumes several times more oxygen per gram of tissue than most other organs, it is exposed to an especially large amount of free radicals; many diseases of the brain, including Alzheimer's and Parkinson's, are believed to involve excessive free radical damage.

We are just beginning to understand the complex relationship between melatonin and the brain. Current research indicates that in addition to sleep disorders and neurodegenerative conditions, melatonin might prove useful in some forms of depression, chronic pain and even schizophrenia.

Melatonin and the Immune System

Both the immune function and melatonin levels decline dramatically with age. Is this merely a coincidence or is there a cause-and-effect relationship? Recent research clearly shows that melatonin has immune-enhancing properties. Suppression of melatonin production in animals creates a state of immune deficiency that is reversed as soon as melatonin levels are brought to normal. In one study, old mice given melatonin, were able to produce twice as many antibodies in response to infection as the control group. In another study, melatonin reduced the mortality of mice infected with encephalitis virus from 100% to 44%. The ability of melatonin to boost immunity is especially pronounced when the immune system is weakened by stress, disease or old age.

Melatonin and cancer

Presumably help from melatonin dates as far back as the Sixties. The first scientific evidence of melatonin's possible anti-cancer activity appeared in the Eighties following experiments in animals and human tissue cultures. In several rodent studies after the administration of potent carcinogens, melatonin fully or partly blocked the development of tumors. Drs.' Blask and Hill showed that melatonin suppressed the growth of the human breast cancer cell line MCF-7 by 75% (these are cells derived from an actual breast tumor sample and then grown in culture).

Amazingly, researchers found that melatonin was effective in about the same range of concentrations that are naturally present in the human body - too little or too much didn't work. This was an effect quite different from what one would expect from an anti-cancer agent. Most chemotherapy drugs become more effective (and more toxic) as dosages are increased. In another study, researchers treated one batch of MCF-7 cancer cells with constant levels of melatonin and another with alternating levels roughly simulating the natural rhythm of melatonin production in the body. The regimen with alternating highs and lows was more effective. Demonstrating the natural pattern of melatonin production is apparently optimal for inhibiting the growth of tumor cells.

We do not know with any degree of certainty, that melatonin supplements can prevent cancer in the human body. Theoretically, melatonin may help counteract two of the factors in the development of cancer: free radical damage and deterioration of the immune system. Animals studies indicate that supplemental melatonin might prevent carcinogenic tumors, but the only way to get a definitive answer in humans is to conduct long-term, large-scale studies, which hopefully, will be done in the near future.

The ability of melatonin to enhance certain cancer treatments and even extend the lives of untreatable cancer victims has been shown in several clinical studies. In a study involving 100 patients with untreatable metastatic tumors, an immunotherapy regimen of low dose IL-2 (an immunostimulant) and 40 mg melatonin daily induced partial tumor regression in 17% of the patients. None of the patients receiving supportive care alone improved. Twenty-one were still alive after one year, but only 5 in 48 in the untreated group lived. In patients with metastatic colon cancer which was unresponsive to standard chemotherapy, the IL-2 plus melatonin regimen produced a partial tumor regression in 3 of 25 treated patients. None of the 25 untreated patients regressed. Survival at one year was significantly better in the immunotherapy group (9 of 25 versus 3 of 25 in the untreated group).

Scientists believe that melatonin exerts beneficial effects in cancer patients through several mechanisms: reducing the rate of growth of cancer cells; stimulating the immune system, particularly natural killer cells to attack cancer; and mitigating stress caused by other treatments and illness itself. As of today, the use of melatonin in cancer therapy is uncommon and largely confined to a few research centers. In the future, however, melatonin may well become a standard item in many cancer treatment protocols.

MELATONIN AND STRESS

As we will see in Part II, old age is in some ways similar to a state of chronic stress. Many scientists believe that the benefits of melatonin are especially dramatic when stress or old age weaken the body. In fact, it may be a part of the body's natural defenses against the deleterious effects of stress. Indeed in several studies, melatonin was shown to prevent gastric ulceration and other damage seen in severe stress. In other studies, stressed and old animals stood a much greater chance of surviving a serious infection when given melatonin.

Melatonin may protect the body from stress through the following mechanisms:

- Prevention of stress-induced immunodepression by stimulating the immune system
- Antioxidant protection from large amounts of free radicals generated by stress
- Preservation of neurons in the hippocampus, the area of the brain important for normal regulation of the stress response
- Stimulation of the release of opioid peptides which play a role in limiting stress response

CHAPTER 7

DHEA: BEATING THE AGING CLOCK

DHEA (dehydroepiandrosterone) is one of a number of hormones which have been widely publicized in recent years. DHEA is actually a steroid produced by the adrenal gland. While this gland produces dozens of steroids, DHEA is the most abundant. DHEA appears to have many important roles in the body. It is used as a precursor for the synthesis of male and female sex hormones. It also acts directly on many organs and tissues to produce a barrage of physiological effects. The levels of DHEA in the bloodstream reach their peak in young adulthood, but it's all downhill from there.

Note: Much of the DHEA circulating in the body (about 90%) is in the form of DHEA sulfate (DHEAS), a derivative of DHEA. DHEAS and DHEA are interconvertible and the former can be considered as the storage form of the latter. DHEA is cleared from bloodstream much faster than its sulfate and its levels swing up and down throughout the day. On the other hand, the levels of DHEAS are rather stable and are a good indicator of overall DHEA production in the body. For that reason, researchers and clinicians often measure either DHEA and DHEAS levels or DHEAS alone.

An increasing number of people believe that restoring youthful levels of DHEA can reverse some aspects of aging and increase life expectancy. Much of that belief is based on numerous animal trials done with DHEA over several decades. DHEA was shown to increase life span in rodents, improve the immune system, and provide some protection against heart disease, diabetes, cancer and other conditions. But as they say, a rodent is a rodent is a rodent.

Unlike humans, rodents have a very low level of circulating DHEA(S) in their bloodstream, which means that their tissue may respond quite differently to higher levels. Thus, animal studies of DHEA are useful in planning human research rather than predicting the effects of DHEA replacement in humans. For this reason, we will abandon these studies in favor of the human clinical studies of DHEA.

Unfortunately, none of the human studies has lasted more than a year. If the story on estrogen replacement is any indication, the long-term effects of DHEA may not be known or fully understood for another 2 or 3 decades. Despite this, indirect evidence indicates that DHEA may play a role in delaying the aging process in humans. There is evidence that high DHEA levels correlate with preserved functional capacity in the elderly whereas low levels correlate with higher risk of heart disease, rheumatoid arthritis, asthma, diabetes and other chronic conditions. One should keep in mind that correlation does not necessarily mean that low DHEA levels contribute to diseases or aging, but may be a consequence or a coincident phenomenon.

DHEA and Immunity

In 1997, researchers at the University of California evaluated the effects of DHEA replacement (50 mg a day for 20 weeks) on the immune system in 9 healthy men whose average age was sixty-three. DHEA replacement significantly increased the number and activity of certain types of immune cells (monocytes, natural killers and B- and T-lymphocytes). An intriguing finding of this study was the elevation of levels of IGF-I, the key mediator of the action of growth hormone. This result suggests that some of the effects of DHEA and growth hormone may go through the same pathway. The researchers concluded that DHEA has potential therapeutic benefits in immunodeficient states.

Current evidence also indicates that DHEA may increase the efficiency of vaccines among the elderly. Vaccinations can sometimes be ineffective in the elderly because their immune systems are too weak for the vaccine to work effectively. For the same reason, the elderly have a much greater chance of dying from an infection than younger people. In one study, a group of elderly individuals over sixty-five were vaccinated with influenza vaccine and given 50 mg of DHEAS for 2 consecutive days. At the same time a similar group was vaccinated without DHEAS. In the DHEAS group there was a four-fold increase in the ability to develop antibodies against influenza virus. Of course, further research is needed to truly evaluate the potential of DHEA as a vaccine enhancer for other infections.

Another promising avenue is the use of DHEA in the treatment of autoimmune diseases, a host of conditions in which the immune system attacks its own body's tissues. The risk of contracting an autoimmune disease increase with age, due in part to age-related changes in the immune system. Presumably, DHEA may help to restore the normal balance of forces to the immune system.

To date, the most promising research has come from the double blind study conducted at Stanford University using 28 female patients with SLE (systemic lupus erythmatosus). SLE is an autoimmune condition occurring predominantly in women and characterized by swollen joints, skin rash, and mouth ulcers. In this study, 200 mg of DHEA a day (versus placebo) improved the overall severity of the disease and allowed a reduction in dosages of drugs. (Typical drugs for SLE are high doses of corticosteroids which produce numerous side effects). Other studies have found a tendency toward low levels of DHEA in such autoimmune conditions as rheumatoid arthritis and multiple sclerosis. It remains unclear whether this is a contributing factor or a consequence of the disease.

DHEA AND THE BRAIN

To date, there is a large enough body of evidence to conclude that DHEA has some direct effect on the brain. The extent and nature of this effect has yet to be determined.

In his 1996 book "DHEA, A Practical Guide", Dr. Ray Shahelian reviewed the conclusions of many physicians who extensively use DHEA in their practice. Most doctors noted that DHEA improved mood and sense of well-being in a majority of patients. Some patients also reported better memory and clearer thinking. A small 1997 study demonstrated that DHEA relieves depression and improves memory. Further research is required to confirm these findings.

Several studies in mice showed that DHEA and its precursor, pregnenolone, improve memory and learning at dosages ten to a hundred times lower than any other neuroactive steroid. Once again, levels of DHEA in rodents are much lower than in humans, which means that the human brain may not be quite as responsive.

DHEA AND HEART DISEASE

Some steroid hormones like estrogens may protect the body from heart disease. Other steroid hormones such as cortisol may do just the opposite. As the production of estrogens ceases after menopause, the occurrence of heart disease in women increases. Some studies indicate that estrogen replacement therapy can lower the risk of atherosclerosis and heart disease in women.

Evidence indicates that DHEA may have a similar effect in men. A large epidemiological study in 1,000 older men and 942 older women provided evidence that DHEA had a slight protective effect against heart disease in men, but not in women. Another study showed that men under age fifty with premature arterial plaque had lower DHEA levels than age-matched men without coronary artery disease.

There's no doubt that DHEA directly affects at least one of the mechanisms involved in heart disease - the formation of blood clots. Clots can attach themselves to arterial walls and block the flow of blood, causing heart attacks. Aspirin, prescribed by many doctors to patients with heart disease works by thinning the blood; i.e., by inhibiting the formation of clots. Studies show that DHEA also slows the formation of clots and speeds up their dissolution.

The effects of DHEA on cholesterol and blood lipids in humans remains unclear. The results of animal studies tend to be either inconclusive or dependent on a particular species: DHEA lowered total cholesterol and LDL levels in monkeys and hogs, yet had the opposite effect in rabbits.

DHEA AND SEX DRIVE

Can DHEA improve sex drive? The jury is still out. At present, there is no clinical data that addresses this issue. One study, however, looking at various effects of DHEA did not find any changes in the patients' libido. On the other hand, Dr. Sahelian, who surveyed hundreds of clinicians treating patients with DHEA, firmly believes that DHEA does boost the sex drive, especially in those with low DHEA levels, an effect which appears to be stronger in women.Theoretically, DHEA may enhance sex drive through two mechanisms: being a precursor of sex hormones, DHEA may stimulate their production; and as a neuroactive steroid, DHEA may activate the central mechanisms of sexual stimulation.

CARBOHYDRATE METABOLISM, DIABETES AND OBESITY

Aging is associated with a progressive loss of tissue sensitivity to insulin, which leads to elevated blood sugar. Mild elevation of blood sugar after meals is called carbohydrate intolerance or prediabetes, whereas an elevation of fasting blood sugar is a sign of diabetes. A large percentage of older people have carbohydrate intolerance and many will eventually develop type II diabetes. In prediabetes and early stages of type II diabetes, the blood levels of insulin are abnormally high because insulin-producing cells try to overcome insulin resistance. Eventually these cells burn out, and full-blown diabetes ensues.

As we mentioned earlier, insulin resistance contributes to several mechanisms of aging as a result of increased blood sugar and insulin levels. Several human studies have shown that DHEA improves the responseviness of tissues to insulin, and therefore, may prevent type II diabetes.

Interestingly enough, the reverse relationship between DHEA and insulin sensitivity also appears to be true. Researchers at Virginia Commonwealth University studied the effects of the drug Benflurolex, which improves insulin sensitivity and reduces insulin excess on the blood levels of DHEA and DHEAS in middle-aged and elderly men. Reduction in insulin excess and blood glucose was associated with an almost two-fold increase in DHEA and DHEAS levels in middle-aged men. In elderly men, the effect was even greater, with DHEAS levels increasing by 167%.

The effects of DHEA on total body weight vary depending on the species and even the strain of animals. Available human data indicates that DHEA does not have any significant effect on body weight. In a 12-month study done with 15 sixty to seventy-year-old women treated with 10% DHEA cream once daily, a slight, yet statistically significant improvement in body composition was observed.

CHAPTER 8

AGING AND IMMUNITY: KEEPING YOUR IMMUNE SYSTEM UP AND RUNNING AFTER YOU START SLOWING DOWN.

Every minute of every day, our bodies are involved in a battle with an enemy that threatens our very existence. It is an army whose weapons are invisible, toxic and sometimes lethal. They are the millions of microscopic invaders we call bacteria, viruses and parasites. They constantly bombard our defenses. They are carried in the air we breathe, the food we eat, the things we touch. Our skin is literally crawling with these potentially deadly pathogenic microorganisms.

Under normal conditions, our immune system is highly efficient. It eliminates any potential threat before it becomes a real danger. Occasionally, however, invaders break through the front lines and start to build up its forces within the body. Then the immune system initiates an intense, aggressive response - fever, aches, pains, soreness, malaise or swelling. In other words, an infection. A healthy immune system usually rids the body of infection within a few days and returns its forces to its "border-patrolling" routine. However, if the immune system is weakened by disease (most commonly AIDS), aging, stress or malnutrition, it leaves the body virtually defenseless. If the immune system is extremely weak, as in the advanced stages of AIDS, even an aggressive antibiotic treatment will ultimately fail.

Today, we know that the immune system is a highly complex and finely-tuned biological "war machine," with specialized subdivisions, intricate communications systems and hierarchy. It employs several types of specialized cells, including lymphocytes, macrophages, and granulocytes, each having its own responsibilities and fighting resources (see Table 3). The key organs involved in producing or

White blood cells	Modes of action	Main functions
Granulocytes	• Phagocytosis	• Engulf foreign organisms
Macrophages	• Phagocytosis • Release of cytokines	• Engulf foreign organisms and present antigens on their surface that help activate lymphocytes • Activate lymphocytes • Suppress appetite • Induce fever and malaise
T-Lymphocytes (cell mediated immunity)		
Helpers	• Recognize foreign antigen and send chemical messages	• Induce response in other T-cells and B-cells
Inducers	• Stimulate T-cell development	• Stimulate immature T-cells in the thymus to develop into mature T-cells
Killers	• Release noxious chemicals	• Destroy invading organisms
Suppressors		• Suppress immune response
B-lymphocytes (humoral immunity)	• Produce antibodies	• Make foreign organisms an easy target for phagocytosis by macrophages or granulocytes • Kill foreign organism directly
Natural killer cells	• Release noxious chemicals	• Destroy cancer cells and virus-infected cells

Table 4. Principal Cells of the Immune System

housing immune cells are the thymus, lymph nodes and spleen. Like any good army, the immune system relies on a sophisticated and efficient communication network. Immune cells can produce special signal molecules called cytokines, which carry messages from the immune cells to other tissue. For instance, some cytokines, such as cytokines interleukin-2 and interleukin-4 stimulate the growth of immune cells, whereas interferons have anti-viral, anti-bacterial and anti-tumor effects.

The immune system in mammals loses its efficiency with age. A weakened immune system also increases the risk of cancer and possibly, atherosclerosis. Infections are the fourth leading cause of death in America. Generally, the more robust one's immune system is, the greater the chances are of living a long life, free of disease.

One of the most dramatic age-related changes the immune system suffers is the shrinkage of the thymus gland. Located behind the breastbone, the thymus is the "training center" for T-lymphocytes, one of the key classes of immune cells. A well functioning thymus is required to keep T-lymphocytes plentiful and active. The thymus is at its largest during early childhood, but as one grows older, it begins to shrink and decrease activity. Actually, shrinkage of the thymus is considered one of the most reliable biological markers of aging.

It is still largely unclear why the thymus shrinks with age which correlates with the decline in growth hormone and melatonin. In animals, removal of the pituitary or pineal gland, which produces GH and melatonin correspondingly, causes the thymus gland to shrink. Treating old animals with GH or melatonin restores the activity of the thymus. It would appear that the deterioration of the thymus gland and the loss of immunity that accompanies it are not inevitable consequences of aging. They can be reversed through the restoration of youthful levels of GH and melatonin.

The immune system is highly dependent on an adequate supply of nutrients, particularly protein, vitamins and trace minerals. Deficiencies of vitamins A, C, E, B complex, folate and pantothenic acid can compromise various aspects of the immune system, and of these, the most common are vitamin A, B12 and folate deficiencies. Zinc deficiency is one of the world's most widely spread nutritional problems. Zinc is one of dozens of enzymes employed by the immune cells. However even a slight deficiency can depress the immune system. Zinc supplements restores the immune function within a matter of weeks. On the other hand, excessive and prolonged supplementation of zinc can result in copper deficiency, which can impair immunity and other functions. Zinc supplement in excess of RDA requirements should not be taken for more than a month. If there is a clinical reason for long-term zinc supplementation, copper should be supplemented as well (at zinc-to-copper ratio 15 : 1 by weight).

Iron deficiency, especially common in infants, menstruating women and the elderly, can also impair immunity. In one study, infants receiving adequate iron and vitamins had 50% fewer respiratory infections than those who received adequate vitamins but were iron deficient.

In the elderly, an adequate diet may not be enough to maintain desirable levels of all vitamins and minerals. Many older people have difficulty absorbing iron and vitamin B12 so that normal amounts of iron and B12 in the diet may still result in a deficiency.

Supplemental vitamins can help prevent age-related decline of the immune system. Vitamin E dramatically improves various aspects of the immunity, particularly the activity of lymphocytes and macrophages. In a number of animal studies, large doses of vitamin E markedly increase survival after severe viral and bacterial infections.

Vitamin A supplements can also improve immunity. However, vitamin A is toxic in high doses and should be used with caution. Doses above 10,000 IU for more than 2 months are not recommended. Pregnant women and children are at a special risk of vitamin A toxicity and should not take supplements exceeding RDA without a doctor's supervision. Contrary to popular belief, megadoses of vitamin C (1-2 grams per day or more) only slightly, if at all, improve the resistance against and recovery from infections. When studies were performed to determine if vitamin C supplements reduce the risk or decrease the duration of the common cold, the results were inconsistent. Even if vitamin C does work against the common cold, the result is probably modest. Vitamin C deficiency, however, is detrimental to immunity and wound healing. Stress or injury increases the requirements for vitamin C and may produce deficiencies with intakes that would normally be considered adequate.

Other nutrients were also shown to affect immunity. The amino acid arginine, taken in significant quantities, improves various immune parameters. For instance, supplementary arginine inhibited the growth and spreading of experimental tumors in animals. Arginine is hypothesized to stimulate immunity by enhancing the release of growth hormone and also directly stimulating nucleic acid synthesis.

RNA or ribonucleic acid consists of chemical units called nucleotides. The body can synthesize these substances, but the rate of synthesis is limited in some dietary sources. In animals, restriction of dietary nucleotides or RNA suppress T-cell function. A balanced diet usually contains plentiful amounts of RNA or nucleotides, and it remains unclear if additional supplementation will stimulate the immune system.

The intake and type of fat in the diet also effects the immune system. The body uses some polyunsaturated fatty acids to synthesize prostaglandins, the chemical messengers involved in inflammation and some immune responses. Levels of prostaglandins are affected by dietary intake of various fatty acids. Diets high in omega-6 polyunsaturated fatty acids, found in abundance in safflower and corn oil, were found to suppress some aspects of the immune system and promote tumor growth. The immunosuppressive effect was especially pronounced when omega-6 polyunsaturated fatty acids were partially oxidized by cooking. Polyunsaturated fats rich in omega-3 fatty acids (fish oil) were shown to improve several immune parameters, including the ability of T-lymphocytes to respond quickly to infection.

In recent years, the connection between the brain and the immune system has been widely documented. In several studies, depression was found to adversely affect the immune system. Notably, the effect of depression on the immune system was proportionally greater as subjects grew older. Treatment for depression usually reversed negative immune changes.

As we will discuss in later chapters, psychological as well as severe

Vitamin	Affects
Pyridoxine (B6)	Impaired lymphocyte response to cell division stimulants Impaired antibody production Impaired T-cell function Decreased activity of the thymus Atrophy of lymphoid tissue
Pantothenic acid	Impaired antibody production
Riboflavin (B2)	Impaired antibody production Involution of the thymus Impaired function of granulocytes (neutrophils) Impaired lymphocyte response to cell division stimulants
Folic acid	Impaired function of granulocytes (neutrophils) Impaired lymphocyte response to cell division stimulants Impaired function of T-killer cells Impaired antibody production
Vitamin (B12)	Impaired lymphocyte response to cell division stimulants Impaired function of granulocytes (neutrophils)
Biotin	Impaired antibody production Impaired T-cell function Atrophy of the thymus
Thiamin (B1)	Modest impairment of antibody production
Vitamin C	Impaired inflammatory responses Impaired function of T-killer cells Impaired phagocytic function of granulocytes an macrophages
Vitamin A	Impaired antibody production Impaired lymphocyte response to cell division stimulants Increased susceptibility to some tumors
Vitamin E	Impaired antibody production Impaired lymphocyte response to cell division stimulants Impaired phagocytic function

Table 5. Effects of vitamin deficiencies on the immune responses (adapted from Modern Nutrition in Health and Disease, 8th edition, 1994, edited by Shils, Olson, Shike)

physical stress have detrimental effects on the immune system.

Immunity and Exercise

Physical exercise has a modest effect on the immune system during youth, but prolonged bed rest or other reduction in physical activity impairs immunity. This causes a decline in the number of white blood cells and reduces the ability to produce antibodies in response to foreign substances.

As the body ages, the beneficial effects of exercise on the immune system increases. One possible reason is that exercise may stimulate the release of growth hormone and IGF-I. At a young age, these hormones are abundant and already exert as much immunostimulation as possible, but in older people, the levels of GH and IGF-I tend to be low and the stimulation of their release may boost the immune system. Another possibility is that exercise improves carbohydrate tolerance and reduces insulin excess, both known to benefit immunity. Again, these parameters are usually normal in young adults but impaired in older individuals.

Autoimmunity

Perhaps the greatest challenge facing the immune system is destroying invaders without harming the body's own cells. The immune system's sophisticated mechanisms discriminate between foreign and native cell substances and selectively destroys interlopers. Although these mechanisms are usually very reliable, they do fail occasionally, resulting in an autoimmune attack (when the immune systems mistakes some healthy organ(s) or tissue(s) for an enemy and attempts to destroy it). The most common type of autoimmune attack is mediated by so-called autoantibodies (antibodies against the body's own cells).

Antibodies are special proteins produced by B-lymphocytes and designed to react with foreign substances. Enemy cells marked by attached antibodies are then gobbled up by macrophages or destroyed by other means. When antibodies-gone-crazy bind to the body's own cells, the damage may be severe. A number of serious diseases are caused by this self-destructive behavior of the immune system, including: rheumatoid arthritis, systemic lupus erythematosis and psoriasis.

While overt, intense autoimmune conditions are relatively rare, mild autoimmune reactions are rather common; their incidence clearly increasing with age. In fact, some scientists view mild-to-moderate autoimmunity as a hallmark of aging. In particular, the elderly tend to have more autoantibodies in their bloodstream. Figuratively speaking, many elderly suffer a mild rejection of their own tissues. Autoimmunity may be a factor in the gradual atrophy of organs with age. Amyloid, a toxic age pigment capable of destroying brain cells, nerves and other vital tissues, is believed to be a by-product of autoimmune reactions.

Why does autoimmunity increase with age? Strangely enough, it may be an indirect consequence of the age-related deterioration of the thymus gland. The thymus produces several kinds of immune cells, including so-called T-suppressors, responsible for keeping excessive and self-destructive immune responses in check. As the thymus shrinks, T-suppressors become less active and therefore less capable of regulating the activity of other immune cells, particularly B-lymphocytes. As a result, more self-destructive B-lymphocytes escape control and begin producing autoantibodies. While acute autoimmune disorders usually require immunosuppressant drugs such as corticosteroids or cytotoxic agents, a somewhat opposite approach, may work in the elderly with mild autoimmunity. Regenerating the thymus may improve the balance within the immune system and reduce autoimmune reactions.

CANCER AND IMMUNITY

There is no doubt that the immune system plays a key role in protecting the body from cancer. It is believed that cancer cells constantly develop in the body, but the vast majority are destroyed by the immune system. Only those cancer cells that escape surveillance give rise to advanced cancers. There has been some success in combining traditional methods of cancer therapy such as radiation, chemotherapy and surgery, with immunotherapy. It is also believed that spontaneous regression of tumors seen in a very small number of patients is due to the activation of the immune mechanisms.

There's little doubt that the risk of cancer dramatically increases with age. It's unclear, however, how much of a role age-related decline of the immune system contributes to cancer growth. Only T-cell immunity suffers severely with age while other aspects of the immune system may remain intact. AIDS patients, who have markedly decreased T-cell immunity, show a dramatic increase in the risk of some cancers, notably Karposi's sarcoma. However, the cancers most often seen in healthy older people (e.g. colon, lung or breast cancer) are not found at increased frequency in AIDS patients and conversely, Karposi's sarcoma is extremely rare in the healthy elderly.

CHAPTER 9

AGING AND DEPRESSION: NEARLY AS COMMON AS THE COMMON COLD

It's now 7:10 A.M. Your clock radio has been blasting for 45 minutes, but you still can't muster the strength to drag yourself out of bed.

After a monumental struggle you manage to hit the shower, wolf down a bowl of cereal and drive to work.

You've reached a point in your life where nothing really matters anymore; job, home life, friends. It seems the only thing you are capable of feeling is exhaustion.

You were supposed to pick up groceries on your way home but you forgot. Your spouse will be home any minute. They'll start chewing your ear off again. You haven't made love in months. What's more, you don't even want to.

If this sounds familiar, there's a good chance that you are suffering from some form of depression. Of course, you may think depression is a character flaw, but it's really a flaw in chemistry - a lack of norepinephrine and serotonin.

Before we explore the link between aging and depression, perhaps you should be familiar with its symptoms:

- Subdued, irritable or anxious mood; physical inactivity or hyperactivity.
- Lack of self-confidence; low self-esteem; self-reproach; inappropriate guilt.
- Loss of interest in usual activities; loss of sexual desire.
- Social withdrawal; detachment.
- Diminished ability to think or concentrate.

- Negative expectations; hopelessness; helplessness; increased dependency.
- Recurrent thoughts of suicide.
- Fatigue; loss of appetite; weight loss, or weight gain.
- Insomnia or hypersomnia; loss of sexual desire.

The presence of 5 or more of these symptoms is a strong indication of depression. Serious depression is not something to be taken lightly. It requires professional help. Nothing we can say here could possibly take the place of sound, professional treatment by a psychiatrist or a psychologist.

Depression is the most common mental problem in our society. It is estimated that about 25% of the population will experience clinically significant depression at some point in their lives, and even more suffer a milder form of depression.

It is important to consider that the incidence of depression dramatically increases with age. In 1996, Dr. J. Haller and colleagues studied a group of 880 Europeans born from 1913 to 1918 and found that 12% of all men and 28% of women were suffering from depression. Other studies indicate that in some areas the rates were far greater.

The relationship between aging and depression is a two way street: the aging process contributes to the development of depression and depression contributes to the process of aging. Before we continue, we need to briefly review the causes and mechanisms of depression.

The human brain is an extremely complex structure containing literally billions of cells. The key brain cells, neurons, are highly complex and capable of varying their behavior depending on the environment. Just as our world today is dependent on reliable, high-speed communications, proper brain function relies on efficient communication between neurons somewhat like our economy depends upon reliable high-speed telecommunications. The nature of interneuronal communication is both electrical as well as chemical. When a neuron "wants" to send a signal to another, it first sends an electrochemical wave along its axon (a microscopic tube-like elongation serving as a communication line). As the signal reaches the end of the axon, it triggers the release of neurotransmitters from the axon's tip into the synaptic cleft (the space between the axon's tip and the body of another neuron). Neurotransmitters are small molecules required for the transmission of a signal from one neuron to another across the synaptic cleft. Key neurotransmitters include norepinephrine, acetylcholine, serotonin and dopamine. The neurotransmitters released by one neuron act on special molecular "push-buttons" (receptors) located on the membrane of another causing it to "feel" the signal and respond with an action. After the signal has gone through, the neurotransmitters remaining in the synaptic cleft are either destroyed by the enzyme monoamine oxidase (MAO) or recaptured by the neurons, and transmission is thus terminated.

Based upon our current knowledge, depression, whatever the underlying causes, occurs when the levels of neurotransmitters are too low, leading to poor communication between neurons. Since norepinephrine and serotonin are especially important in mood regulation, most drug treatments of depression are aimed at raising the brain levels of one or both of these neurotransmitters.

Many things can precipitate or trigger depression. Some people are genetically predisposed to depression and usually develop depression early in life, requiring extended professional care. The most frequent cause of depression, however, is acute or chronic psychological stress caused by a myriad of circumstances including the loss of a loved one, divorce, lay-off, financial troubles, work-related stress, etc.

Normally, the body's response to stress is self-limiting. At the onset of stress, the hypothalamus signals the pituitary to release ACTH (adrenocorticotropic hormone), one of the key molecules involved in the body's response to stress. ACTH, in turn, stimulates the release of stress steroids such as cortisol from the adrenal glands (many of the effects of stress on tissue are mediated by stress steroids). The rise in the blood levels of stress steroids causes the hypothalamus to turn off its initial signal, and the stress response gradually subsides. However, during prolonged periods of stress, the hypothalamus becomes less sensitive to negative feedback from stress steroids. It appears that this is achieved via the reduction in the levels of neurotransmitters in the brain. In other words, prolonged stress tends to shift our brain chemistry closer to that of depression. The reverse is also true: in depressed patients, levels of stress steroids are often elevated and the mechanism that limits the stress response is impaired. In many ways, depression is a state of prolonged, self-perpetuating stress.

Diseases associated with, chronic pain and immune or hormonal disturbances, are also serious contributors to depression. Most people with chronic pain have some degree of depression. Nutrient deficiencies can also result in depression, in particular, deficiency of vitamins B1, B6, B12, C, folic acid, niacin and pantothenic acid - usually (but not always) along with a host of other symptoms. Overt deficiencies of these nutrients are uncommon in developed countries but marginal deficiencies may be common, especially in the elderly and chronically ill and may contribute to a large proportion of cases of depression.

There are important physiological similarities between depression and the aging process. Firstly, levels of neurotransmitters in the brain, including norepinephrine and serotonin decrease with age. As mentioned earlier, low levels of neurotransmitters are the most prominent feature of depression. Second is the impairment of the feedback mechanism necessary for limiting an excessive stress response, which results in a state of chronic stress.

Thus, aging appears to contribute to depression by shifting the body's biochemistry. However, the reverse relationship also exists. Depression appears to accelerate aging and increase the risk of disease through several mechanisms:

(1) Depression leads to excessive stress. Psychological changes in depression resemble those seen in chronic stress. Depression leaves a person much more vulnerable to all sorts of acute stress. While a healthy person can overcome personal crisis with minimal psychological consequences, a depressed individual may plunge in a prolonged, self-perpetuating life crisis, (in itself a form of serious stress). Stress, as we discuss in Part II, accelerates aging by intensifying essentially all its mechanisms.

(2) Depression adversely effects the immune system. It is not quite clear how depression impairs immunity, but there's no doubt that it

clear how depression impairs immunity, but there's no doubt that it does. It was found that some neurotransmitters stimulate the immune system and a lack of these molecules would seem to be a factor in impairment. Excessive production of stress steroids seen in many depressed individuals is also detrimental to the immune system. Since the immune system provides protection from infections, cancer, atherosclerosis and may shorten the life span, impaired immunity can increase the risk of disease.

(3) Depression accelerates the central aging clock. This is the hypothesis of V. Dilman, author of the neuroendocrine theory of aging or "the central aging clock theory." According to Dilman, the central aging clock works through reducing the sensitivity of the hypothalamus to negative feedback, thereby causing a variety of changes in the body. The clock's "mechanism" appears to involve a slowdown in the production of the levels of neurotransmitters in the hypothalamus and some adjacent brain structures. Since depression also reduces levels of neurotransmitters, it may accelerate the central aging clock. Dilman suggested that all antidepressants that raise the levels of neurotransmitters in the hypothalmus are potential anti-aging drugs. There is no direct evidence that definitively proves this theory. However, in many studies it was found that drugs or nutrients that relieve depression tend to shift the body's metabolic and adaptive characteristics to a "younger" pattern and may extend life. In particular, the antidepressant *deprenyl* was found to increase life span in rats by 34%. It also reduced lipofuscin accumulation and neuron degradation in the brains of rats.

(4) Depression decreases motivation, preventing a person from actively pursuing the goal of life extension or even maintaining a basic healthy lifestyle.

Treatment of depression often combines two distinct approaches, counseling, designed to improve a patient's view of their life situation and coping with problems, encouraging positive activities and social interactions. The other approach, is to correct biochemical imbalance in the brain by raising the levels of neurotransmitters.

There are numerous drugs designed for this purpose, but they most-

rons to recapture neurotransmitters after the signal has gone through - more neurotransmitters are then left in the synaptic cleft, which somehow improve interneuronal communication and relieves depression. The best known drugs of this kind are **Elavil** and **Prozac**. Elavil blocks recapturing of norepinephrine and serotonin. Prozac blocks the reuptake of serotonin only. Another important class of antidepressants is monoamine oxidase inhibitors which reduce the activity of the enzyme that destroys neurotransmitters. Again, the result is an increase in the levels of neurotransmitters in the space between neurons which eventually reverses the depression.

Unfortunately, most antidepressants have significant side effects including sedation, constipation, dry mouth, nausea, stomach upset, lightheadedness, impotence and others. For this reason, drug treatment is usually reserved for clinically significant depression. Some nutrients and food supplements can also help increase the levels of neurotransmitters in the brain and thus improve depression and they tend to have fewer side effects.

CHAPTER 10

SEXUALITY AND AGING: LOVE IS A MANY SPLENDORED THING, EVEN AT 70

Sex is as essential to life as breathing itself. In terms of priorities, having a normal, enjoyable sex life is second only to physical survival. Even that is somewhat questionable depending upon whom you ask. From an evolutionary standpoint, the drive to procreate must be extraordinarily powerful to ensure the survival of the species.

As a society, we are consciously and subconsciously bombarded by sex from all sides. It influences the way we dress, what we read, the way we think. Sex has literally permeated our culture, even our economy. Today, commercials selling the most asexual products like chewing gum are permeated with sexual themes and overtones.

Although sexual drive (libido) and capacity decrease with age, loss of sexual activity does not have to be an inevitable consequence of aging.

The current view among many scientists and clinicians reveals that sexual relationships can and should positively contribute to life enjoyment and self-esteem at any age. In their review of sexuality in old age, Drs.' Comfort and Dial from the University of California, state that "aged individuals need sexually and medically what people in general want and need, and the idea of an acceptable decline into a sexless state is insulting."

In laboratory animals, it's easy to study the impact of aging on sexuality simply because there are fewer variables to complicate the issue.

However, it's relatively difficult to conduct truly reliable studies on sexual behavior in people, particularly those past their youth. Firstly, they're often reluctant to participate. Secondly, the sample is usually biased in one way or another. Thirdly, the most common research methods rely on truthful answers to a questionnaire.

Nonetheless, it is clear that in many older people sexuality is alive and well. In general, individuals who have preserved their health tend to retain a robust sexual function. However, many age-related disorders contribute to a decline in sexual activity. Atherosclerosis, diabetes, prostate enlargement and hypertension are detrimental to male sexual function, where depression can suppress libido in both men and women. The drugs commonly used to treat these conditions can cause impotence and inhibit sexual desire. Another major cause of decreased sexuality is stress. Biologically, it's quite understandable: stress diverts resources from such functions as digestion and reproduction to those critical for immediate survival. (We'll discuss this in greater detail in Part II).

MENOPAUSE AND ESTROGEN REPLACEMENT

Menopause is the cessation of the monthly menstrual cycle in women, occuring when the ovaries stop producing estrogens. On average, menopause occurs at age fifty, but it may occur as early as a woman's late thirties.

When estrogen levels drop, female reproductive organs lose their functionality. In particular, the walls of the vagina become dry, irritated and often infected, making intercourse a painful, unpleasant experience. Since regular intercourse is itself a factor in maintaining normal vaginal lining and lubrication, avoiding intercourse because of irritation often exacerbates the problem.

Along with the onset of menopause, women tend to experience a host of symptoms during the first 2 to 5 years: hot flashes, fatigue, insomnia and nervousness.

Today, the most common treatment for menopause is estrogen replacement - to reverse the atrophy of the reproductive organs and eliminate or reduce hot flashes and other symptoms.

Estrogens are not just sex hormones: they can directly affect most organs in the body, including the brain, heart, blood vessels, lungs and bones. The effects of estrogens on the body are numerous. However, estrogen replacement has its benefits and its drawbacks.

Can the upside of estrogen replacement outweigh the downside? Most studies indicate that it slightly reduces overall mortality and improves the quality of life in women. The most comprehensive study to date, conducted by Dr. Francine Grodstein in Boston, sampled 121,000 women on hormone replacement for 16 years, from 1976 to 1992. Researchers found that estrogen replacement significantly reduced overall mortality by 37% for 10 years and by 20% for more than 10 years. Improved survival was largely due to the lower mortality rate from heart disease and stroke. On the other hand, women who took estrogen for more than 10 years had a 43% increase in the risk of breast cancer. The study concluded that women with risk factors for heart disease stand to gain the most from estrogen replacement. These risk factors include a family history of heart disease, cigarette smoking, hypertension, high cholesterol and obesity. Women with a low risk of heart disease, but an increased risk for breast cancer should probably avoid taking estrogens, especially for more than 10 years.

The decision to initiate estrogen replacement therapy should be made on an individual basis by a woman and her physician, taking into account medical history, concerns and individual preferences. According to Dr. Grodstein, "women and their doctors should re-evaluate that decision every 5 years or so because the risks and benefits change over time." Those who opt to refrain from estrogen replacement can maintain vaginal lubrication through use of topical estrogen-containing creams or, to avoid even small doses, use water-soluble lubricants.

Sex drive and the ability to experience arousal are well preserved in many, if not most, postmenopausal women in spite of the loss of ovarian function and substantial atrophy of the reproductive organs. On the other hand, some women lose much of their libido after menopause. The reasons for this variation is not quite clear. Some tissues other than the ovaries, such as adrenal glands and fat tissue, can produce small but significant amounts of estrogens, which may have a role in maintaining sex drive. It was also found that testosterone is not only important in the sex drive among men but in women as well. Functioning ovaries produce small amounts of testosterone, about 1 to 2 mg per day, but after menopause, the only remaining source of testosterone is the adrenal glands which may not produce testosterone in sufficient quantities to maintain a healthy sex drive. Indeed, in some postmenopausal women with decreased libido, estrogen replacement proves ineffective. However, when a small amount of testosterone is added to the regimen, sex drive is often restored.

Supplementing testosterone in postmenopausal women, however, should be done very carefully because of the risk of virilization; the appearance of male features, such as facial and body hair growth, lowering of voice, etc. Postmenopausal women not on estrogen replacement therapy are at special risk because estrogens, which normally counteract some effects of testosterone, are at relatively low levels.

Can menopause be postponed?

In humans, menopause is an inevitable consequence of aging and cannot be avoided. However, there is an extremely wide variation in terms of its onset.

We're just beginning to understand why some women remain fertile relatively late in life. One possible explanation is the pace of the ovarian biological clock. The function of ovaries is two-fold: to produce sex steroids, mainly estrogen needed to maintain the function of female reproductive system, and to prepare mature follicles (special cells ready for fertilization with sperm) from precursor cells called oocytes. Every woman has a limited number of oocytes and can produce only a limited number of mature follicles. Sequential cycles of ovulation deplete the reserve of oocytes, the ability to ovulate is lost and menopause occurs. It is believed that this depletion of "ovarian capital" somehow causes the decline in estrogen production and shrinkage of the ovaries seen in menopause.

However, there is evidence that the initial number of oocytes in ovaries are not the only factor in forecasting when menopause will occur. During each cycle, many oocytes begin to develop into mature follicles. Only one (or rarely few) complete the journey, and the remainder degenerate and die. If many oocytes are "pushed into the race" at each cycle, the reserve will be depleted more quickly leading to early menopause. Yet if only a few oocytes are used up per cycle, the woman's fertility may be preserved longer. It appears that the rate of depletion of oocytes is affected by the central aging clock in the brain's hypothalamus, which regulates the function of ovaries by causing the pituitary to secrete the hormones called gonadotropins, **luteinizing hormone** (LH) and **follicle stimulating hormone** (FSH), which stimulate ovulation and estrogen production. The mechanism of the central aging clock (discussed in Chapter 2) is such that gonadotropin levels increase with age. During puberty, the increase of gonadotropin levels helps to switch on the reproductive function, but later it simply causes excessive stimulation of ovaries and speeds up the depletion of ovarian reserves. Some researchers believe that slowing the pace of the central aging clock may reduce ovarian depletion and delay menopause.

One way we can reset the central aging clock is by increasing the levels of dopamine in the hypothalamus to make it more sensitive to feedback signals. Dophaminergic stimulants, such as L-DOPA or bromocryptine, were shown to restore menstrual cycles in old laboratory animals and some postmenopausal women. At present, the extension of a woman's reproductive life into the sixth or seventh decade is based upon a modest amount of data and promising theory, but perhaps, in a few decades a sixty-something-year-old mom may move from the CNN's story-of-the-year to an everyday occurrence.

MALE SEXUAL FUNCTION

Following young adulthood, men experience a steady decline in sexual function. This becomes increasingly obvious after age fifty. These age-related changes in male sexuality are dubbed **male menopause**, although not as dramatic as female menopause.

The causes and contributing factors in male menopause remain the subject of heated debate, but the most obvious candidate is the decrease in testosterone levels.

Starting in the fourth decade of life, testosterone levels usually decrease at a rate of about 1% yearly. Chronic disease, stress and drugs may increase that rate. In most healthy older men testosterone levels remain in the normal range and the correlation between testosterone levels and sexual activity is little or non-existent. Many studies indicate that testosterone replacement is likely to improve the sexual function of men with low testosterone levels (below 300 ng/dl, the lower boundary of the normal range) and will occasionally benefit older men with normal testosterone. Also, testosterone replacement will often increase muscle mass and may reduce body fat. A possible downside of testosterone replacement includes the suppression of testicular function (both less testosterone and less sperm is produced), acne, worsening of hypertension, and mild suppression of the immune function. The consequences of long-term testosterone replacement in older men are unknown. Our current body of knowledge suggests that among those who show testosterone levels within the normal range, replacement of DHEA may provide the same benefits as testosterone in terms of body composition and libido, but with fewer side effects.

THE GAP BETWEEN LIBIDO AND POTENCY

Although men tend to retain an interest in sex as they grow older, their ability to perform often suffers. The result called the **libido-**

potency gap, is a highly frustrating situation where sexual desires sometimes exceed physical capacity. The incidence of impotence increases dramatically with age. While 90% of men under fifty are physiologically potent, only about half of those over seventy are.

Until recently, impotence was thought to be the result of mainly psychological factors. While low self-esteem and other psychological factors may exacerbate the problem, it is now believed that about 75% of these cases have physical (organic) causes. In older men, organic impotence is even more prevalent, amounting to about 90%.

Impotence is medically defined as an inability to achieve an erection sufficient for sexual intercourse. Erections are achieved by a coordinated effort of several systems in the body: circulatory, nervous, endocrine (hormones), and genitourinary (prostate). To put it simply, an erection depends on "plumbing" and "neurological wiring" being in good working order. An appropriate signal sent through the nerves causes penile arteries to dilate and veins to constrict. As a result, the inflow of blood into the penis is greater than the outflow, causing an erection. Adequate levels of testosterone and some neurotransmitters, such as norepinephrine, are important in maintaining the wiring necessary to produce an erection. A healthy prostate is also important because prostatic disease may cause compression of arteries and nerves at the base of the penis, which, in turn, can lead to impotence.

CAUSES OF IMPOTENCE

Insufficient arterial blood flow is probably the most common cause of impotence and is usually the result of atherosclerosis, hypertension, or diabetes. Significant atherosclerosis (blockage of arteries by fatty deposits) is extremely common in men aged thirty-five to forty and can be completely asymptomatic. Impotence is only one of the many dire consequences of atherosclerosis, which include heart attacks stroke, etc. High blood pressure can mechanically damage and harden arteries as well as promote atherosclerosis progression. Diabetes can cause impotence by damaging both large and small blood vessels as well as the nerves.

Venous leakage increases inflow of blood via arteries into the penis is necessary, but not sufficient for erection. The veins should also be able to contract to help hold more blood in the penis. Hence, some cases of impotence are caused by excessive venous leakage during erection.

Impaired nerve supply damage to the nerves that regulate blood flow to the penis can be caused most commonly by diabetes, as well as pelvic trauma and some diseases of the nervous system.

Drugs and alcohol, many medications (high blood pressure drugs, antidepressants, sedatives, even some over-the-counter drugs) as well as alcohol, can cause impotence. Discontinuing the drug, if possible, usually cures the impotence. Sometimes an alternative drug with the same benefits, but without adverse effects on sexual potency can be found.

Diseases of the prostate two very common prostate conditions - benign prostate enlargement, seen in men after age forty, and prostatitis, seen in men of all ages, can result in impotence by compressing arteries and nerves at the base of the penis and, sometimes by simply producing pain in the area. Radical prostatectomy (complete surgical removal of the prostate) often leads to impotence, potentially because the nerves that control erection are severed.

Hormonal imbalance impotence is due to hormonal imbalances in particular, low testosterone and ocassionally high prolactin in a relatively small number of cases. Psychogenic impotence is more common in young and middle aged men than in older men. It is estimated that about 25% of cases of impotence have a psychological origin. If a man has a spontaneous erections while asleep or upon awakening, then impotence is likely to be psychogenic. Psychological stress and/or anxiety may be interfering with the signals that the brain sends to peripheral nerves in a sexually arousing situation. As a result, peripheral nerves fail to normally regulate the blood flow in and out of the penis. Also, a long-term psychological stress may upset the body's hormonal balance, lowering testosterone and elevating prolactin. Thus contributing to psychogenic impotence.

For all its varied causes, organic impotence is usually the result of one or more age-related diseases. Atherosclerosis, the most common cause of impotence, can be prevented and partially reversed when cholesterol and LDL are substantially lowered through diet, exercise, nutrient supplements and in refractory cases, cholesterol-lowering drugs. The best strategy against diabetes is prevention or early treatment geared towards improving the responsiveness of tissues to insulin. Mild hypertension can be improved through a diet high in potassium, calcium and magnesium, while severe cases usually respond to medication. Unfortunately, some blood pressure medications may themselves cause impotence. BPH is a condition believed to result from age-related hormonal changes, particularly the increase in the conversion of testosterone to its derivative **dehydroptestosterone** (DHT). Some degree of BPH is found in the majority of older men. The enlarged prostate may obstruct the flow of urine, causing urinary frequency and urgency. Penile arteries and nerves are compressed by BPH and DHT, leading to impotence. Again, it should be stressed that a comprehensive life extension strategy would help prevent or forestall these age-related diseases and reduce the risk of impotence even in advanced old age.

About 25% of all cases are the result of psychogenic impotence. The percentage of cases of psychogenic impotence are considerably higher in younger men because the they are less likely to have organic diseases as well as stable monogamous relationships. Various forms of stress are the most common causes of psychogenic impotence. Enhancing stress resistance with adaptogens, in particular, ginseng extract, was shown to cure or at least improve psychogenic impotence in some men.

THE LARGEST SEX ORGAN

There is little doubt that the human brain is the largest and by far the most important sexual organ. Arousal and orgasm are controlled by the brain through the signals it sends and receives from peripheral nerves. The brain's ability to support sexual activity depends on the presence of sufficient levels of key neurotransmitters. Almost any serious psychiatric disorder can lead to the loss of sexual desire. The most formidable "enemy" of healthy sexuality is depression, especially the type marked by anxiety. Depression is associated with a variety of biochemical shifts that inhibit desire and reduce performance. This includes low levels of some neurotransmitters, such as norepinephrine and serotonin, as well as an excess of stress hormones. As noted, many features of depression are similar to a state of chronic stress. As we age, we are more likely to suffer from depression, often without knowing it. What we may consider a "normal" age-related loss of sexual desire may be a result of latent depression. Once the depression is treated, the sex drive is often "miraculously" revived.

Age-related deterioration and damage to the brain - its most severe forms include stroke, Alzheimer and Parkinson's disease which may impair, and in some cases, destroy sex drive. The brain is highly susceptible to free radical damage because of its intensive metabolism and high content of unsaturated fatty acids, which easily react with free radicals. Antioxidants, especially those which protect neuronal membranes, such as vitamin E and lipoic acid, may slow the aging of the brain and help preserve a healthy sex drive. A "smart nutrient" dymethylethanolamine (DMAE), is known to improve brain function in humans. In animals, DMAE was shown to increase life span and reduce the deposits of age pigments in brain cells. The principal action of DMAE is to increase brain levels of the neurotransmitter acetylcholine. While DMAE does not affect sexual activity in young people, it was reported to increase sex drive in many people after forty. Future research may show the beneficial effects of other neuroactive nutrients or drugs on sex drive in older people.

SEXUALITY AND "FOUNTAIN-OF-YOUTH" HORMONES

Three hormones were praised by the media for their numerous alleged anti-aging and disease-fighting benefits - **growth hormone** (GH), **dehydroepiandrosterone** (DHEA) and **melatonin**. These same hormones decline dramatically with age. Current research indicates that each of these hormones, while not a cure-all, may produce a number of positive changes in older animals and humans.

What can these "fountain-of-youth" hormones do to enhance our sex life? Comprehensive clinical studies of the direct effects of GH, DHEA and melatonin on human sexuality have not been conducted. Most evidence is anecdotal, indirect or purely speculative.

In their 1997 book "Growing Young with GH," Dr. Ronald Klatz and Carol Kahn review the opinions of several clinicians who treated their patients and themselves with GH injections. According to the authors, GH may dramatically improve sexual drive and performance in older people. Theoretically, GH might stimulate sexual function by improving mood and brain function, enhancing cardiovascular performance and altering levels of some hormones, including testosterone.

The effects of DHEA replacement on sexual function need further study. Surveys of clinicians experienced in administering DHEA show that it may stimulate libido, especially in men with low testosterone levels and women. In one study, 50 mgs of DHEA for 3 month did not have any effects on the patients' libido.

The effects of melatonin on sexual function are even harder to assess. Very high levels of melatonin may inhibit sexual function. Melatonin levels are very high in childhood prior to sexual maturation, and their subsequent abrupt decline may act as a trigger to puberty. In literature, some cases of delayed puberty in humans have been linked to excessively high melatonin levels. However, very low levels of melatonin may have negative effects on sexual function in adults. As melatonin deficiency seems to increase the risk of atherosclerosis, high blood pressure and some age-related brain disorders, maintaining youthful levels of melatonin might be a factor in preserving potency and sex drive by reversing these conditions. Melatonin has been hypothesized to slow or even reverse the central aging clock and thereby rejuvenating many body systems. There is already some evidence that melatonin may rejuvenate the reproductive system. Israeli researchers showed melatonin to prevent age-related decline in testosterone levels in rats. The animals treated with the hormone produced almost 3 times as much testosterone as their untreated counterparts.

In Chapter 29 we discuss practical options for revitalizing one's sexual function. Taking steps to reduce the decline in sex drive and capacity over the years is an important part of preserving a healthy and productive lifestyle.

CHAPTER 11

CENTENARIANS: GETTING PAST THE FIRST HUNDRED YEARS.

One day, saying that he had known Pontius Pilate in Jerusalem, he described minutely the governor's house and listed the dishes served at supper. Cardinal de Rohan, believing these were fantasies, turned to the Comte de Saint-Germain's valet, an old man with white hair and an honest expression. "My friend," he said to the servant, "I find it hard to believe what your master is telling us. Granted that he may be a ventriloquist; and even that he may make gold. But that he is two thousand years old and saw Pontius Pilate? That is too much. Were you there?" "Oh, no, Monsignore," the valet answered ingenuously, "I have been in M. le Comte's service for only four hundred years."

— Collin de Plancy, *Dictionnaire infernal* [Paris, Mellier, 1844, p. 434]

Studying humans is no small undertaking. Studying aging in humans is virtually impossible. Most of our knowledge comes from animal experiments employing essentially identical animals fed a well defined diet and living in a controlled environment. Yet the results obtained in animal experiments, especially mammals, have considerable relevance to humans for a number of reasons. Genetic and biochemical differences among species are relatively small compared to the differences in their appearance or behavior. Genetic overlap between humans and mice is over 90%, and between humans and primates, about 98%. When studying a particular body system or a biochemical pathway, scientists usually can select a species in which this system or pathway is much the same as in humans. Decades of medical research have demonstrated that well-conducted and carefully interpreted animal studies are indispensable in advancing our knowledge of the human body.

However, animal studies provide an indirect and somewhat inaccurate understanding of human aging. Although the main mechanisms of aging appear to be similar in all higher organisms, the contribution of each corresponding mechanism may vary considerably. In addition, some systems of the human body and the central nervous system in particular, are significantly different from their animal counterparts. Even in similar systems (e.g. the immune system), subtle differences may have a radically different role in the aging process. The most dramatic example of the limitations of these animal studies is caloric restriction. When rats and mice are fed severely restricted diets starting prior to sexual maturity, their life span can increase as much as to two-fold. In fact, food restriction is the single most effective method of life extension in rodents as well as many other species. In monkeys, however, severe caloric restriction initiated before maturity causes brain damage, shortens life span and malnutrition as well as in humans, too.

Confronting the limitations of animal studies, researchers are now turning to the longest surviving people for new insight into human longevity. Maximum life span in humans is about 120 years but very few live past the age of one-hundred. These 100+ "supersurvivors" called **centenarians**, are now the focus of life extension research in many countries. The proportion of centenarians in overall population has been steadily rising over the past few decades. In the Eighties, the centenarian population grew by 160% in the United States.

According to the 1980 census, about one in 10,000 lives to be over 100 in the U.S.

What is their secret? What do these centenarians have in common? First, they are diverse and scattered; thus obtaining accurate information and history is often difficult. This is partly the reason for disagreement among scientists as to the factors that are critical to super-longevity. It is clear, however, that no one single factor is the key. Extreme longevity is rather the result of a complex interaction of genetic, physiological, environmental (nutrition, lifestyle, etc.), psychological, and social factors. It would be easier to explain the complexities of quantum mechanics to the average 5th grader than to clearly determine the role of each and every factor in long life. However, below is a summary of current views on human longevity based upon the study of the oldest of the old.

1. Genetic factors At the time of this writing, no gene has directly been linked to human longevity. The most likely candidates appear to be the genes involved in DNA repair and protection from free radicals. Centenarians may have unusually active versions of some of these genes. The genes that guide the rate of the organism's development may also affect life span. Yet another possibility is that centenarians have a smaller number of "bad genes," that is, the genes that confer susceptibility to diseases. An example of such a scenario is the gene coding for apolipoprotein E (apo-E), which was shown to be linked to an increased risk of Alzheimer's disease. There are three versions of apo-E gene: E2, E3 and E4. Individuals with E4 have the highest risk of developing Alzheimer's disease and those with E2, the lowest. Researchers found the E4 version of the apo-E gene in 25% of people younger than twenty-five, but only in 14% of those over eighty-five. Such a difference could be a result of the increased risk of death from Alzheimer's disease in those with the E4 version. It is likely that many other genes have several variants which differ in their capacity to confer susceptibility or provide protection against degenerative-diseases.

Several studies indicate that longevity tends to cluster within families, thus supporting the role of genetics.

2. Nutrition There are only a handful of studies related to nutrition in centenarians. Dr. Mimura and colleagues studied dietary patterns in 88 of the oldest people in Okinawa, Japan. The population has the longest documented average life span in the world today. The diet was mostly rice, potatoes, fish and abundant vegetables, well-balanced in vitamins and minerals. The incidence of atherosclerosis is low. Another study found that Okinawans consumed a higher proportion

of animal protein (including fish, milk, eggs, and meat) higher than the national average. Intakes of calcium, iron, vitamins A, B1, B2 and C were also higher.

A study conducted at the University of Georgia compared dietary habits of 24 centenarians with those of the "younger" elderly. The centenarians ate breakfast more regularly, avoided weight loss diets and large swings in body weight. They also tended to eat more vegetables. A larger European study of 6,000 centenarians found that the oldest of the old generally consumed a balanced diet based on natural foods, including plenty of fruits and vegetables.

Overall, the nutritional patterns shared by most centenarian studies includes generous protein intake, and an abundance of fruits and vegetables. Centenarians tend not to consume excessive calories, but their diets are not necessarily low in fat.

3. Metabolism Data on the metabolic characteristics of centenarians is scarce. The most consistent finding is generally good carbohydrate tolerance and responsiveness of the tissues to insulin. A study among Italian elderly, conducted by Dr. G. Paolisso and colleagues, found that carbohydrate tolerance in centenarians was as high as in adults under fifty, and even higher than in old people aged seventy-five to one-hundred. As we previously mentioned, carbohydrate tolerance declines with age in most people. This appears to have an effect in several mechanisms of aging. Poor responsiveness of tissues to insulin causes insulin excess and high blood glucose, both of which contribute to the aging process. It is unclear why centenarians tend to have unusually normal carbohydrate metabolism. One possible explanation is a slower-than-average pace of the central aging clock. Other possible factors include diet and low levels of stress.

4. Psychology and coping ability A group of researchers who studied 96 centenarians in Georgia, wrote that their subjects were "optimistic," wise individuals and very engaged in daily living." A general consensus among gerontologists is that centenarians tend to have an above average coping ability and are successful in quickly overcoming psychological stress. Positive moods and stress resistance may help extend life by maintaining an active immune system, boosting the

release of growth hormone, and slowing down the central aging clock. The biochemical basis for such "mind-over-matter" phenomenon may lay in the link between positive moods and the levels of neurotransmitters in the brain, particularly the levels of dopamine in the hypothalamus. Although not yet quantifiable, this view is supported by abundant evidence that depression, which is associated with low levels of neurotransmitters, accelerates aging and promotes degenerative-diseases. Scientific data aside, it stands to reason that if you plan to increase your life span, you may as well be in the mood to enjoy it.

5. <u>Lifestyle</u> There seems to be no universal lifestyle associated with super longevity. Centenarians are found in many cultures and socio-economic groups, in urban and rural areas, in different climates and geographic zones. The most consistent findings about their life-styles include a comfortable and familiar environment in daily life, a good support network and active engagement in work combined with enough rest. The bottom line would appear to be a low level of stress, which, we believe, is an important key to the secret of outliving your peers.

It is truly awesome when someone approaches or exceeds the age of one-hundred. Yet even more awesome is the fact that centenarians appear to be as healthy or, in some cases, even healthier than their seventy to eighty year-old counterparts. A large European study showed that the oldest old tend to have well-preserved immune systems, especially in the activity of natural killer cells important in cancer prevention, a normal lipid profile, including low cholesterol and LDL, a normal or only slightly impaired carbohydrate tolerance, and a good degree of mental self-sufficiency. Drs. E. Beregi and A. Klinger studied 280 Hungarian centenarians and found them to be healthier than average sixty to eighty year-olds, with lower prescriptive drug use and better adaptive ability. The study of the oldest of the old of the Palau Islands, conducted at the University of California, found that physical and functional mental illness was infrequent, with the most common illness being arthritis.

The evidence of good health in centenarians does not seem to agree with the idea that disease and infirmity increase with age. This is not necessarily a contradiction. Centenarians are not typical - although their numbers are on the rise, they still account for less than 1/10 of 1% of the population. In a majority of people and animals, the aging mechanisms accelerate with time, and converge to cause degenerative-diseases and progressive loss of adaptive capacity and vitality. Centenarians may be the exceptions in whom some aging mechanisms are much slower, which results in longer preservation of health.

You could say that centenarians have lucky genes. But how can this knowledge help the rest of us - those who have "regular" genes and the typical rate of aging. For one thing, centenarians clearly demonstrate that successful aging is possible and the later years can indeed be enjoyable and full of life. Another important finding in centenarian studies is that genetics, although important, is only one part of the picture. It is true that some people with "lucky genes" may live to be a hundred without much extra effort. Most of us have flaws in our genetic makeup. We can increase our chances for long life through a diligent life extension strategy. The less genetically "gifted" an individual is, the more important making proper choices in diet and lifestyle become. To assess your genetic endowment, just look at longevity and health in your family tree.

Here are some examples of how an average person can become "physiologically similar" to a centenarian if they are willing to work at it.

Some centenarians appear to have lower levels of free radicals because their genes encode unusually active free radical-scavenging enzymes. Average people can take antioxidants and nutrients that stimulate the activity of these enzymes.

Centenarians tend to have good carbohydrate tolerance and a high responsiveness of tissues to insulin. In most elderly, however, the situation is quite the opposite, which contributes to essentially all mechanisms of aging. Most of us can normalize our carbohydrate tolerance and insulin response through diet, nutrient supplements, moderate exercise and stress reduction.

Some of the most common traits among centenarians are optimism, a positive mood and a constructive view of life. This is almost the exact opposite of depression, which is almost an epidemic in our society and particularly, among the elderly. There are many nutrients and natural plant extracts that can readjust brain biochemistry, improve your mood and coping ability, and relieve the symptoms of depression (see Chapter 9).

There's far more to the equation of becoming a centenarian than "good" genes, a strong support system, moderate exercise and daily activity. What we have here is a rough outline of several key factors that centenarians have in common. The best way to find out if you are a candidate is by first seeing your family physician.

PART II

CHAPTER 12

EVERYTHING YOU'VE ALWAYS WANTED TO KNOW ABOUT STRESS BUT WERE TOO STRESSED OUT TO ASK

Stress has become one of the most important issues of our time. Almost everything we do involves some degree of stress. We suffer on-the-job stress, financial pressures, social obligations and stress in our personal relationships. There are deadlines to meet, expectations to live up to and tremendous constraints on our time. What's more, even some of our greatest pleasures produce stress. When we root for our favorite team in a close contest, guess what all that fun and excitement produces. Stress. Action thrillers and horror movies are not just simply exhilarating to watch. They're also stressful.

Even though stress accounts for such a large part of our daily lives, people understand very little about it. Most people think that stress is a state of mind associated with tension, anxiety and discomfort. This is only partly true. First and foremost, stress is a scientific concept concerning an organism's interaction with its environment. To truly understand the role of stress in aging and disease, we will need to study it as a physiological phenomenon.

Living organisms survive by maintaining an extremely complex and delicate internal equilibrium called **homeostasis**. In the most general terms, stress is a threat to our inner physiological balance and a threat to our biological status quo. Numerous internal and external forces, or **stressors**, can disturb or threaten our homeostasis. The result, in plain English, is stress.

Stressors take many forms - heat, cold, infection, toxins, injury, pain and strong emotion. Adaptation, in this case, is the ability to successfully overcome, neutralize or avoid stressors. Whenever stress occurs, it triggers a cascade of biological changes collectively known as general adaptation syndrome (GAS) or a **stress response**. Its biological goal is to counteract the stressor and restore homeostasis. However, a paradox exists in that an excessive stress response may itself inflict severe damage to the body, causing disease and accelerate aging.

The idea that successful adaptation to various threatening forces can help maintain the body's delicate equilibrium was around since the days of Hippocrates, the forefather of modern medicine. He believed that disturbing the forces that produced the disharmony of disease were of natural, rather than supernatural origin. During the Renaissance, Thomas Sydenham suggested that the adaptive response to disharmony caused by disturbing forces could itself cause disease. At the turn of the Twentieth century, Walter Cannon described the reaction of emergency as the **fight or flight response**.

Yet without a doubt, the most profound insight into the biological nature of stress was made by Canadian physiologist Hans Selye. According to Selye, stress sets in motion a specific chain of physiological reactions (general adaptation syndrome or stress response), which are essentially the same regardless of the nature of the stressor. In other words, it doesn't matter whether you are hot, cold, injured, sick, overworked, scared, intoxicated or infuriated: your body will generate essentially the same stress response. It's simply trying to adapt to the situation.

The Evolution of Stress

Our physiological response to stress was shaped in a far different environment than the world we live in today. Life for primitive man was filled with hardship and imminent danger in the form of predators, hunger, wounds, infections and extreme variations in weather. To survive this hectic life style, a potent and quick stress response was mandatory. Prehistoric man was not concerned with his IRA or retirement plans. His concerns were more immediate. They revolved around survival, often at the expense of overstraining and wearing down the body.

Today's environment is also filled with stress, but of a totally different nature. We are constantly bombarded by information, social pressures and a world changing so rapidly, it's a daily race to keep up with it. We constantly try to adapt and adjust. The problem is that our adaptive machinery is still basically the same as it was tens of thousands of years ago. Our stress response is still best suited for fleeing wild beasts, enduring intense heat or extreme cold than being stuck on a highway during rush hour.

The stress response is still essential to life. If your car hits a tree or you fall from a second floor window, your body's stress response is your best tool for immediate survival. The same goes for any trauma, infection, surgery or any other life-threatening situation. However, in the vast majority of cases, the stress response is set off when there is no serious threat to survival. For example, making a public speech sets off pretty much the same physiological reactions as our ancestors running from a saber-toothed tiger.

The stress response is simply the body in overdrive mode aimed at overcoming adverse situations. Stress can do considerable harm to the body, but in a life-or-death situation, it can be invaluable.

Unfortunately, the way we evolved as a species, we often generate an intense stress response when there is little or no need for it; i.e., when there is no threat to life or health. This leads to an accelerated depreciation of the body's resources and an increased risk of disease. In other words, stress leads to poor health and accelerates aging.

Ideally, one would want the best of both worlds - to have an efficient stress response during emergencies as well as the ability to avoid the activation of the stress response when there is no real danger. The mechanisms of the stress response, however, are set for emergencies only. The key players in the stress response are the hypothalmus, the pituitary gland, the sympathetic nervous system and the adrenal gland.

THE HYPOTHALMUS AND PITUITARY

The hypothalmus and pituitary glands are responsible for regulating the stress response. The hypothalmus located in the brain's control center is responsible for a wide variety of physiological functions including the stress response. When the hypothalmus senses a stressful situation, it activates the sympathetic nervous system (see below) and also sends a chemical message via a hormone called CRH (corticotropin releasing hormone) to the pituitary gland, a bean-sized structure located near the center of the brain. In response to this message, the pituitary sends a hormone called ACTH, or **corticotropin** to the adrenal glands which in turn, release a barrage of stress hormones (see below).

THE SYMPATHETIC NERVOUS SYSTEM

The sympathetic nervous system is responsible for the regulation of certain involuntary actions such as heartbeat, digestion and sweating as well as other functions. In the initial phases of the stress response, symptoms such as anxiety, quickening of the heartbeat, palpitations and coldness are due to the activation of the sympathetic nervous system. The actions of the sympathetic nervous system on various organs is mediated by the neurotransmitter, norepinephrine.

THE ADRENAL GLAND – "MIDDLE MANAGEMENT" OF THE STRESS RESPONSE SYSTEM

Using a corporate personnel chart as an analogy, the adrenal glands would fall under the heading of "middle management" in the stress response. They secrete key stress hormones responsible for changes in the stress response. The adrenal gland located just above the kidneys consist of two distinct parts: the adrenal medulla and the adrenal cortex.

The medulla, the inner portion of the adrenal gland, secretes two hormones, **epinephrine** (adrenaline) and **norepinephrine** (noradrenaline) collectively referred to as **catecholamines**. These two hormones, along with the sympathetic nervous system play an important role during the alarm phase of the stress response (see below). They produce numerous physiological effects directed at preparing the body for an immediate action: a faster, more forceful heartbeat, quicker respiration, elevated blood glucose, increased muscle tone and heightened alertness. In some people, the release of adrenaline in the initial phase of the stress response produces mild euphoria and is perceived as an enjoyable experience. This is one reason why some people are thrill seekers. In a manner of speaking, adrenaline "junkies" who put themselves in danger to produce this euphoric side effect are "addicted" to the alarm phase of the stress response.

The cortex, or outer portion of the adrenal glands, is very different from the medulla, producing a different group of stress hormones called **stress steroids** (gluccocorticoids). The principal stress steroid in humans is cortisol.

When large quantities of stress steroids are released, they exert a profound effect on the body, raising blood glucose by producing a state similar to diabetes. Stress steroids also suppress the immune system. Overall, the purpose of stress steroids are to boost the body systems vital in emergencies, particularly the central nervous system and cardiovascular system, by providing them with more fuel (glucose and fatty acids). Too often, this comes at the expense of less essential tissue, such as muscle or skin which are partially used for fuel. These massive releases of stress steroids are similar to the body declaring a state of war, but if the system is to survive, no sacrifice is too small. Unfortunately, in many cases, greater amounts of stress steroids are released than needed for health and survival, and as a result, the system may break down because its defenses exact too great a toll.

THE THREE PHASES OF THE STRESS RESPONSE

The stress response is divided into three distinct phases: **alarm reaction, resistance reaction** and **exhaustion.**

THE ALARM REACTION

You are about to ask someone out on a first date. As you approach, your heart races, your feet get cold and you feel nauseous. What if the answer is "No," or worse: "Sure, but I'm busy tomorrow night...and Friday too..." You break out in a sweat, your heart is pounding. No, you're not experiencing a cardiac episode. You're merely experiencing a mild-to-moderate case of an alarm reaction, the initial phase of the stress response.

Sometimes, this phase is justifiably called a "fight or flight" reaction - preparing an immediate physical action by mobilizing the body's resources. The alarm phase is initiated in the brain and involves the activation of the sympathetic nervous system and the release of both adrenaline and noradreneline from the adrenal medulla.

In this phase, the organism's systems are switched to emergency mode, resources are mobilized and the capacity of several key organs and tissues are increased. The hypothalamus signals the pituitary to release corticotropin, which, in turn, causes the adrenals to release stress steroids. All these events facilitate the development of the second phase of stress: the resistance reaction.

THE RESISTANCE REACTION

The alarm reaction is usually brief. The resistance acquired in the alarm phase helps the body to continue to fight the stressor. Stress steroids released by the adrenal cortex play a major role in the resistance reaction. They cause the conversion of lean tissue into energy, elevate blood glucose and suppress everything from inflammation to cell growth. The lean body mass is gradually dwindling.

If the action of the stressor continues, the resistance (adaptation) developed by the organism is eventually lost. Sufficiently intensive or prolonged action of a stressor inevitably leads to the third phase - exhaustion.

Exhaustion

In some situations, the body can undergo successful adaptation to a stressor, enabling it to withstand the stressor without having to maintain a stress response. In this event, the stressor ceases to be a stressor. A person who travels to high altitudes, for example, would initially suffer from hypoxia (low oxygen levels) and develop a stress response. Over several days, the body would produce enough new red blood cells to increase the oxygen-carrying capacity of the blood, and completely offset the hypoxia. The stressor is thus eliminated and the stress response subsides without severe consequences.

There are times when the body is unable to adapt successfully to the stressor and the stress response. The organism's ability to keep up in this "overdrive mode" is limited and sooner or later the resistance reaction gives way to exhaustion. The body's vital functions decline; the resistance of the organism is below its initial level; the body's antioxidant reserves are depleted and there is a loss of body mass and lean tissue. The loss of potassium may cause severe disturbances in the nervous system and in the heart function. The levels of stress steroids may be very high. Conversely, the adrenal cortex may be so overworked, it can't continue producing stress steroids (the latter scenario may cause a dramatic drop in blood pressure, profound hypertension, low blood glucose and general collapse). The blood levels of epinephrine can drop enough to induce a state of shock. Exhaustion caused by a prolonged, intensive stress can be potentially fatal.

In 490 B.C. the Greeks had defeated Persia in a battle on the Plain of Marathon. Legend has it, a Greek warrior, Pheidippides, ran 26 miles to Athens to bring the news of Greek victory. Soon after the good news, Pheidippides collapsed and died. This is a classic example of a fatality caused by the exhaustion phase of the stress response.

How then, does the professional long-distance runner survive a marathon? Stress adaptation: marathon runners have successfully adapted themselves to long-distance races. Their muscles use oxygen and fuel more efficiently, their hearts have greater pumping power and soon for them, a marathon is a medium-strength stressor that elicits a moderate stress response. For an untrained person though, such an effort places a tremendous stress on the body and is potentially fatal.

When Selye studied the stress response in rats, he found that three visible phenomena occurred during the exhaustion phase, now known as Selye's triad: (1) **hypertrophy** (enlargement) and hemorrages in the adrenal cortex; (2) damage to the immune system, including a marked shrinking of the thymus gland, lymph nodes and spleen; and (3) **peptic ulceration**. We now know that essentially all body systems suffer from stress to some degree. The systems vital for immediate survival, such as the nervous system, heart and blood vessels, suffer from overstrain, while other systems are being deprived of nutrients or even dismantled for fuel. Organs already weakened by disease or aging are especially vulnerable and are likely to be the first to break down.

For instance, an elderly patient suffering from pneumonia has a much greater chance of dying from heart failure brought on by combined stress and atherosclerosis, than by pneumonia.

Alarm reaction (fight or flight)

- The sympathetic nervous system is activated; epinephrine (adrenaline) and norepinephrine (noradrenaline) are released from the adrenal medulla.
- The heart rate and the force of the heart contractions increase to provide more blood to organs necessary for immediate survival; blood supply to the skin and internal organs is reduced, except to the lungs and heart.
- The rate of respiration is increased to provide more oxygen for the brain, heart and muscle.

- Blood glucose is markedly increased as the liver breaks down glycogen (a storage form of glucose) and releases the glucose into the bloodstream.
- Digestive activity is halted as nonessential for immediate survival.
- Muscle tone and mental alertness are increased to achieve a heightened readiness for action.
- Perspiration is increased to lower body temperature.
- The stimulation of the adrenal cortex to release corticosteroids is initiated.

Resistance reaction

- The fight or flight reaction has abated and the body has developed resistance to the stressor.
- Stress steroids in blood levels are high and the adrenal cortex continues to produce stress steroids in above normal amounts.
- Blood volume is expanded due to the retention of sodium and excretion of potassium. Blood pressure may be elevated and there is an excess workload on the heart and blood vessels.
- Blood glucose and free fatty acids are elevated, providing extra fuel for the vital systems.
- Proteins from lean tissue, especially the muscle, skin and bone are broken down for fuel; the mobilization of free fatty acids (FFA) from fat tissue is increased - FFA serve as an alternative fuel for most tissues, increasing the availability of glucose to the nervous system.
- The liver produces large amounts of glucose from the amino acids obtained through the breakdown of lean tissue (gluconeogenesis).
- Cell division, protein synthesis and tissue regeneration is suppressed throughout the body as nonessential.
- The immune system and inflammatory responses are suppressed.
- Loss of calcium from the bone is accelerated.

Exhaustion

- The ability to resist stressors is below the initial level.
- Destruction of vital tissues.
- Decline or failure of all or some body systems or organs.
- The hypertrophy and pathological changes in the adrenal cortex.
- Damage to the immune system; involution of the thymus gland, lymph nodes and spleen; destruction of the lymphocytes.
- Depletion of antioxidant reserves.
- Peptic ulceration
- Levels of stress steroids are either very high, or - if the adrenals are damaged - very low.
- The levels of epinephrine and norepinephrine may be very low.
- Hypertension, low blood glucose, shock and death may occur.

Note: Profound exhaustion outlined here occurs only after prolonged severe stress or moderate stress in a very old person; moderate stresses common in life can also lead to significant but less pronounced exhaustion.

Stress in our lives

Severe and prolonged stress is the physiological equivalent of being in a war. It can lead to profound exhaustion, disease or possibly death. Most of us, may never experience such extremes. The stresses we experience are usually mild to moderate, and the occasional severe stresses, such as surgery or major trauma are mitigated by hospital care. Nonetheless, even mild or moderate stress, especially if prolonged, is usually damaging to the body even if it may not cause immediate disease or death, but it will accelerate all aspects of the aging process and increase the risk of disease.

PHYSICAL VERSUS EMOTIONAL STRESS

The stress theory divides stress into two main categories - physical and psychological. Physical stress is caused by factors such as infection, radiation, trauma and severe extremes in temperature. Humans can also initiate a stress response without suffering actual damage. When the central nervous system analyzes a situation and perceives a need for emergency measures, it triggers the stress response immediately. When you spot a mugger lurking at a bus stop late at night, the ability to set off the stress response can be a true lifesaver.

Emotional stress can be just as potent as physical stress. In rodents, overcrowding or prolonged isolation produces a very strong stress response. In humans, stress can be caused by an almost infinite variety of emotional and social conflicts or tensions. To act as a stressor, an emotionally charged event does not have to bear a direct relationship to the individual. For instance, fans watching a sporting event frequently develop some degree of stress response.

Although the triggering mechanisms for both physical and emotional stress are inherently different, the stress response itself is largely the same and both types accelerate aging and impair resistance to disease.

In the civilized environment of the Twentieth century, the impact of stress on our daily lives has shifted from physiological to psychological. Modern man faces a different type of jungle than our ancestors. This one that makes our lives less physically taxing, but more psychologically frustrating than life was even twenty years ago. This is due to technological advances like air-conditioners, elevators and a myriad of other things that put less strain on our physiology.

However, psychological stress exacts an extremely heavy toll. Each day we are faced with a blitzkrieg of information. We live in a society in which we can change spouses almost as easily as we change jobs. Our kids are being raised by a "surrogate parent," MTV. Everything seems out of control. Life is clearly more hectic, competitive and demanding. Drs. T. Holmes and R. Rahe developed a social readjust-

	Life event	Score
1	Death of spouse	100
2	Divorce	73
3	Marital separation	65
4	Jail term	63
5	Death of a close family member	63
6	Personal injury or illness	53
7	Marriage	50
8	Job termination/loss	47
9	Marital reconciliation	45
10	Retirement	45
11	Change in health of family member	44
12	Pregnancy	40
13	Sex difficulties	39
14	Gain of a new family member	39
15	Business adjustment	39
16	Change in financial state	38
17	Death of a close friend	37
18	Change to different line of work	36
19	Change in number of arguments with spouse	35
20	Large mortgage	31
21	Foreclosure of mortgage or loan	30
22	Change in responsibilities at work	29
23	Son or daughter leaving home	29
24	Trouble with in-laws	29
25	Outstanding personal achievement	28
26	Wife begins or stops work	26
27	Beginning or end of school	26
28	Change in living conditions	25
29	Change in personal habits	24
30	Trouble with boss	23
31	Change in work hours or conditions	20
32	Change in residence	20
33	Change in schools	20
34	Change in recreation	19
35	Change in church activities	19
36	Change in social activities	18
37	Small mortgage	17
38	Change in sleeping habits	16
39	Change in number of family get-togethers	15
40	Change in eating habits	15
41	Vacation	13
42	Christmas	12
43	Minor violation of the law	11

Table 6. The social readjustment rating scale developed by Holmes and Rahe. Stressful events are rated according to their potential to instigate disease. A score of 200 per year is considered to be predictive for serious disease.

ment scale, a widely accepted method for rating the levels of psychological stress (see Table 4). A cumulative score of 200 or more in a year is believed to indicate a high risk of developing a serious disease.

Good and bad stress

All men may be created equal, but all stresses are not. Prolonged or excessive stress can overstrain the body's vital systems and deplete its resources. Needless to say, this type of stress is anything but good, leading to a shorter life span and higher risk of disease. However, there's another form of stress that's harmless and potentially beneficial, called mild or moderate short-duration physical stress. In many ways, it stimulates several of the body's adaptive systems, ensuring better resistance. This kind of stress is not intense enough or prolonged enough to produce any appreciable damage; i.e., a vaccination.

In animal studies, periodic exposure of rodents to mild doses of radiation or toxins made them more resistant to larger doses as well as other stressors. However, there is a much more suitable physical stressor that's perfect for improving general adaptive capacity and stress resistance, exercise. The health benefits of exercise are well documented and include improved cardiovascular function, lower cholesterol and LDL, raised HDL, reduced blood pressure, relieving anxiety and aiding in depression. In other words, exercise improves both the psychological and physical ability to cope with stress. The mechanism of anti-stress action of the exercise include the following:

- A short term increase in free radicals during exercise which induces a prolonged increase in the capacity of free radical-scavenging systems.
- Tissues are more sensitive to insulin and improvement in the metabolism of carbohydrates and fats.

- Stimulation that releases growth hormone in young and middle-aged individuals which has many anti-stress and anti-aging properties.
- Reduction of the intensity of "fight or flight" reaction in response to psychological stress.
- May improve the efficiency of the hypothalamic feedback loops, thereby improving the efficiency of the systems that limit the stress-response.

At the time when our stress response "machinery" was still being formed, vigorous physical action was the most common response to emotional stressors: fear prompted flight - anger provoked fighting. In stressful situations, physical activity also plays a role in the feedback mechanism. It limits the intensity of the stress response and produces a calming effect. Although our physiology has remained unchanged since primitive man, our behavior under stress has changed considerably. Emotional stress does not often require escape or fight, and the stress response is more intense and prolonged than necessary for the situation. For that reason, exercise can be especially beneficial during psychologically stressful times.

As with most things, too much of anything can do more harm than good. You can overdo exercise and actually achieve a result opposite to your goals. Excessive exercise, especially without enough rest and adequate nutrition is a serious stressor that can deplete antioxidant reserves, overstrain the cardiovascular system (especially in persons with heart problems) and lead to exhaustion. Any high intensity exercise program should be done in conjunction with an adequate diet containing enough calories and protein to prevent the loss of lean tissue as well as antioxidants to neutralize the increased levels of free radicals. Some dieters engage in excessive exercise while restricting their consumption of calories, protein, vitamins and antioxidants. This approach rarely reaches the goal of lasting weight loss, but often causes profound exhaustion, loss of vital tissue, malnutrition and other problems.

While moderate periodic short-term physical stress is often beneficial, the same does not appear to be true for emotional stress. Occasional short-term emotional stress, such as an exam or public appearance, is relatively harmless. On the other hand, frequent emotional stresses, such as everyday marital fights or high-pressure jobs tend to merge into a state of chronic stress leading to accelerated aging and disease.

CHAPTER 13

STRESS AND THE MECHANICS OF AGING

Once again we bring up the name Hans Selye. Not simply because we admire his work or that we're thinking of starting a fan club, but as the father of the modern stress theory he was the first to suggest that stress actually accelerates aging.

It's never been more apparent that stress is a critical factor in the rate of aging. In addition, stress is considered a key factor in the development of age-related diseases. Studies indicate that animals who are hyperactive to stressful situations have a shorter life expectancy. The most consistent and perhaps most remarkable feature in centenarians is their ability to cope and quickly overcome psychological stress.

Hyperactivity to stressors may give some survival advantages to an animal living in the wild. But, in a relatively stable environment, whether a zoo or some concrete jungle, over-responsiveness to stress can be hazardous to your health.

This doesn't mean that a weak stress response isn't equally or potentially more harmful. In the world we live in today, there is an occasional need for a robust stress response. Surviving accidents and infections, enduring rigorous exercise, the daily commute, weather extremes and night shifts (no kidding) require a reasonably potent stress response. A small amount of stress hormones are required for just normal day-to-day existence, even without emergencies. In fact, some people have no stress response such as those having a rare condition called Addison's disease that is characterized by the failure of the adrenal cortex to produce cortisol and other stress steroids.

Untreated, Addison's disease can be fatal. Treatment is based on daily supplementation with stress steroids. A patient suffering from Addison's disease who has an infection or some sort of trauma is given additional amounts to simulate a normal stress response.

The point is that the stress response is essential and we do need it - so long as it's optimized for a given situation. A weakened response allows physical stressors to damage the body. Conversely, an overly strong response can be harmful. An excessive stress response is much more common than a weak one.

Most of today's stressors are psychological and evoke an unnecessarily potent stress response. As we age, the body's ability to regulate the stress response declines, and our body is less able to shut down the stress response when no longer required. Studies show that the elderly often release more stress steroids in response to a stressor than younger individuals.

The bottom line is that life extension and disease prevention both require an optimal stress response. For the vast majority of people and situations, this means that the stress response should be mitigated - both by avoiding severe or prolonged stress and by modifying the response to it.

Stress and free radicals

Free radicals are highly and randomly reactive by-products of cellular respiration while they have a key role in the aging process. Free radicals are constantly being produced in every cell of the body.

In simple terms, the more calories we burn, the more free radicals we generate. Species with a higher metabolic rate (i.e., those who burn lots of calories per amount of tissue) tend to have shorter life spans. In laboratory animals, caloric restriction reduces both metabolic rate and free radical levels, increasing life span up to two-fold. Free radicals have also been implicated in the development of many diseases from atherosclerosis and arthritis to cancer and cataracts.

Reducing free radical damage is critical to life extension and disease prevention.

Stress dramatically increases the number of free radicals in the body. The main goal of the stress response is to increase the capacity of the systems vital to survival - the nervous system, the cardiovascular system, the lungs and the muscles, achieved by supplying the cells with more fuel (mainly glucose and fatty acids) and stimulating them to produce more energy. One of the side effects of this shift into high metabolic gear is an increase in the production of oxidation by-products, or free radicals.

When you view your body as a machine, you begin to realize the true magnificence of its design. For instance, its stress response has a built-in mechanism to offset the increase in free radicals. This is accomplished through the activation of the antioxidant system. There is evidence that stress hormones can scavenge free radicals, but the organism's antioxidant resources are limited and can be overwhelmed by intense or prolonged stress that generates a flood of free radicals.

Several types of free radical damage are seen during serious stress. Cell membranes suffer most because they contain lipids rich in polyunsaturated fatty acids which are especially vulnerable to free radical attack. Significant free radical damage to biological membranes make them rigid and leaky, detrimental to the cell's normal operations. In particular, leakage in the cell membranes of mitochondria, the cell's "power stations," lead to a precipitous decline in energy production. Normally, when mitochondria burn fuel, they produce the biological equivalent of energy called ATP (*adenosine triphosphate*). Leaky mitochondria however, are poor energy producers; they burn fuel uselessly generating an overabundance of free radicals instead of ATP. Cells with dysfunctional mitochondria are starved despite the abundance of fuel and become overwhelmed by free radicals because, lacking ATP, the repair system is out of order due to a lack of ATP.

Another grave danger from free radical damage is the leakage of **lysosomes**. Lysosomes are little membrane sacks containing a host of potent digestive enzymes used for recycling cellular waste.

When free radical damage causes lysosomes to leak, digestive

Stressor	Malonic aldehyde in relative units
Control (no stressor)	100
Suspension by a skinfold for 24 hours	610
Intoxication (oxidized oleic acid 4 ml/kg)	380
Immobilization for 17 hours	286
Three day fast (without thirst)	241
Burn	205
Hyperthermia at 39-40 $^{\circ}$C for 6 hours	188
Swimming with load (6% of body mass) for 90 minutes	188
Cold exposure, 0 $^{\circ}$C for 24 hours	161
Hypodynamia	147

Table 7. Accumulation of malonic dialdehyde in mice in various stressful conditions. Malonic dialdehyde is an indicator of free radical damage.

enzymes spread throughout the cell's interior chopping up vital cellular structures, including DNA. Finally, free radicals can cause leakage in the cell's outer membrane causing the intracellular electrolytes and proteins to leak out allowing the extra cellular fluid to leak in. Needless to say, this upsets the balance of vital biochemical reactions. Free radicals can also directly damage DNA and proteins. The latter can be replaced, but some DNA damage may be irreversible.

Cells continuously exposed to excess free radicals lose their vital functions quickly and their aging clocks tick faster. Specifically, the cells exposed to high levels of free radicals reach the limit of cell divisions (Hayflick limit) faster and accumulate more unrecycled molecular garbage (age pigments). Such cells are also more likely to turn cancerous because free radicals are potent mutagens that increase the risk of cancer- inducing DNA lesions.

All in all, serious stress can generate enough free radicals to inflict some irreversible damage upon body tissue. It can even kill certain cells, leading to faster aging and increased risk of disease.

Substances that protect us from free radicals can also reduce stress-related damage. In rodents, stress ulcers can be prevented with large doses of various antioxidants. Vitamin E and some synthetic antioxidants reduce stress-related damage to the immune system. In a sense, antioxidant supplements work better during stressful periods than they do in easier times. When you take antioxidants in a completely stress-free environment, your own antioxidant systems may become "lazy" because they sense the arrival of outside help. On the other hand, during serious stress, your antioxidant defenses are already maxed out, so antioxidant supplements are an extremely valuable reinforcement, not a substitute.

For comprehensive protection from free radical damage, it is important that both fat and water-soluble antioxidants be included. Vitamin E, for instance, protects cell membranes and lipoproteins in the plasma. Water soluble antioxidants, such as vitamin C and cysteine, protect DNA and most proteins. Lipoic acid and melatonin are special in that they are both soluble in water and therefore protect all biological structures.

An effective way to boost the capacity of your own antioxidant systems is exercise. Exercise appears to "train" your antioxidant defenses. Moderate exercise causes a short-term elevation in free radical levels to stimulate the production of free radical scavenging enzymes. The levels of these enzymes tend to remain high even long after exercising, and provides extra protection from free radicals. This is somewhat similar to building up one's resistance to poison by carefully taking very small doses.

Adaptogens are yet another weapon in fighting free radical damage. Many adaptogens (e.g., Siberian ginseng) reduce stress-related free radical damage by both mitigating the stress response and stimulating the body's antioxidant defenses.

STRESS AND THE CENTRAL AGING CLOCK

By now you're probably well aware that the human body has a central clock pacing the rate of development and aging. A variety of things influence the pace and stress is no doubt one of them.

As we discussed in chapter 2, the pace of the central aging clock depends on the efficiency of communications between the hypothalmus and the rest of the body. In particular, when the hypothalmus is highly responsive to feedback from organs, the central aging clock's pace is slower.

Evidence indicates that stress has a profound impact on the brain and the hypothalmus in particular. The effects of stress on brain cells include increased free radical damage, an accelerated accumulation of age pigments and even death of brain cells. All of this can contribute to the speeding up of the central aging clock. One particular finding is that stress appears to gradually damage the system that limits the stress response, thereby making the response to future stresses progressively more excessive. For example, the efficiency of the body's stress limiting system partially depends on the **hippocampus**, a structure in the brain functionally linked to the hypothalmus. Damage to the hippocampus impairs the ability of the brain to shut down the stress response when it's no longer needed. It was found that stress steroids can directly damage the hippocampus and lead to an excessively intense and prolonged response to stressors.

Stress also affects the central aging clock by elevating blood glucose. The stress response induces a diabetes-like state in the body, characterized by high blood glucose and decreased responsiveness of tissues to insulin. It is not entirely clear how, but this also tends to accelerate the central aging clock.

Stress and cellular clocks

Most of the cells in higher organisms have a limited ability to divide and grow. As the number of divisions reaches its limit (the Hayflick limit), the cell can no longer divide, accumulates age pigments and loses some of its functionality. On average, the Hayflick limit is about 50 divisions, but this number is not carved in stone. It can be extended or foreshortened by a number of factors. High levels of free radicals shorten the Hayflick limit. Although there are no direct studies to corroborate this, it is likely that the flood of free radicals unleashed by serious stress may shorten the Hayflick limit in many tissues.

Stress, glycation and cross-linking

Glucose is ubiquitous in foods and always present in the bloodstream. It is one of the primary fuels of the nervous system, and essential to sustaining life. Unfortunately, glucose is an ally that can sometimes turn into an enemy, randomly reacting with vital cellular structures like proteins and DNA, altering their properties and functions. Even worse, glucose enables cross-linking, a process in which abnormal chemical bridges form between biological molecules. Cross-linking is among the major causes of cataracts, atherosclerosis, hypertension, and loss of elasticity in the skin and joints. The rate of cross-linking is markedly increased by free radicals.

Stress creates the perfect environment for glycation and cross-linking because it elevates blood glucose and generates large amounts of free radicals.

Stress and age pigments

Some of the waste produced by our metabolism is not eliminated, remaining in the cells in the form of age pigments. They are large insoluble clumps of molecular garbage that can impair normal cell activity and eventually suffocates the cell completely. Free radicals are the main cause of the accumulation of age pigments. Stress causes a dramatic rise in the level of free radicals and leads to faster accumulation of age pigments.

Aging and stress: A vicious cycle.

As we age, many of our organs begin to lose their efficiency. Our heart pumps less vigorously. Our reflexes slow down. Our hearing and vision become less acute. Even our minds become less responsive and agile. In light of this, it would be only natural to suppose that the intensity and vigor of the stress response also declines with age.

Oddly enough, quite the opposite appears to happen. Several key aspects of the stress response actually become more intense. The same exact stressor tends to evoke a greater response in older animals and humans than in younger individuals. In simple terms, this means the stress response actually becomes progressively more excessive with age. In fact, older individuals often show elevated levels of some stress hormones even in the absence of stress. This is the equivalent to living in a chronic state of stress. It's a vicious cycle: stress accelerates aging and aging increases stress.

There has been much research on how aging affects stress. Studies show that older animals respond to stress differently than younger ones in the following ways:

- Older animals produce more stress steroids in response to the same stressor.

- After the stressor is no longer present, older animals continue to have elevated levels of stress steroids and other stress hormones for longer periods of time.
- Older animals produce abnormally large amounts of stress steroids, even in the absence of a stressor, i.e., with a congenital condition.

All these findings appear to hold true for humans as well, although individual results vary significantly. The elderly tend to produce excessive amounts of stress steroids under stress and may have elevated levels of stress hormones, even under normal conditions. This means that older people not only tend to have an abnormally strong and possibly damaging stress response, but may also be in a state of

Signs and Symptoms	Aging	Cushing's disease
Body composition shifts towards more fat and less lean tissue. Body fat is redistrubuted: faces become rounder, the torso becomes fleshier, especially at the abdomen, while the amount of fat in the legs diminishes; the Skin is thin and atrophic with poor wound healing and easy bruising	Common	Typical
Muscle wasting and weakness	Common	Typical
Hypertension	Common	Typical
Osteoporosis	Common	Common
Glucose intolerance	Common	Common
Psychiatric disturbances	Common	Common
	Relatively common (mainly depression)	Common

Table 8. Similarities between some of the normal signs of aging and Cushing's disease. In both, there is an excess of cortisol, the main stress steroid produced by the adrenal cortex.

chronic stress, even in the most pleasant environment.

There is an amazing similarity between certain symptoms of aging and a condition called Cushing's disease, a condition in which the adrenal glands produce excessive amounts of stress steroids, simulating a state of perpetual stress. Of course, aging and Cushing's disease are not thesame. In aging, an excess of stress steroids is due to an excessive stress response. In Cushing's disease, overactivity is due to the abnormality of the pituitary or adrenal glands. Nonetheless the similarities between aging and Cushing's disease appear due, at least in part, from the same cause - excess stress steroids, particularly cortisol.

It is still not entirely clear why the elderly tend to develop hypersensivity to stress and/or remain in a chronic state of stress. The main cause appears to be the disturbance of the brain-to-body connection responsible for curtailing the stress response when it has fulfilled the need. Somehow, the brain doesn't seem to recognize the point when the stressor is neutralized or unnecessary, and fails to call off the stress response. According to the central aging clock theory, this is the result of an age-related impairment in the ability of the hypothalmus to respond to all kinds of feedback signals, including those needed to shut down the stress response.

CHAPTER 14

STRESS AND ADAPTATION

In a sense, living organisms have a love-hate relationship with their environment. On one hand, it provides the essentials needed for survival, such as water, food and the oxygen we breathe. On the other hand, environmental changes can create a deadly threat through exposure to extreme cold, heat, food shortage or predators. Human life on earth has evolved through our innate ability to adapt to an ever-changing environment.

Our bodies are remarkably equipped with the ability to adapt based upon millions of years of evolution. Even in a reasonably civilized environment, we constantly need to adapt to change. In most cases, we don't even realize adaptation is taking place. Our metabolism, for instance, adapts to seasonal changes in temperature by altering the production of thyroid hormones. Our brain adapts to new jobs and new types of activities by learning and creating new reflexes and habits. Our immune system adapts to the continuous onslaught of pathogenic microbes by generating specific, tailor-made antibodies against the invaders.

Our adaptive capacity peaks at about age twenty and then starts to decline. In fact, the loss of adaptability is the principal feature in aging and is one of the main causes of death in later years.

Pneumonia and influenza very rarely kill young people, however, they are the 5th leading causes of death in the elderly. When extreme heat or cold strikes, the victims are almost invariably older people.

Although some loss of adaptability with age is inevitable, the degree of loss varies considerably. Adaptability is best preserved in those individuals who retain close to optimum response to stress and a high degree of functional capacity of their vital organs.

Adaptation has two principal stages: (1) general adaptation syndrome or stress response, and (2) adaptation to a specific stressor.

When a stressor of any kind is encountered for the first time, the body responds with a standard emergency reaction and the stress response. The goal of the stress response is two-fold. First ensure the functioning of the systems vital to immediate survival and second, provide plentiful resources to the organs and systems involved in the specific adaptation to the stressor. For that purpose, the body suppresses nonessential functions, like digestion and immunity and partially breaks down nonessential lean tissue for fuel and building blocks. The freed resources are then redirected to enhance the activity of the key survival systems and also of the systems required for adaptation to the stressor. In time, specific adaptation to the stressor develops and the stress response subsides.

A familiar example of this two-stage process is exercise. In a person not used to strenuous exercise, an unusual exertion provokes a full-blown stress response, including the release of large amounts of epinephrine (adrenaline) and stress steroids. The person experiences extremely rapid heartbeat, palpitations, nausea and other symptoms of acute stress followed by general malaise and exhaustion. If this person continues regularly exercise, the body begins to adapt to the new requirements. Heart and skeletal muscles enlarge and become stronger and more fuel-efficient, lung capacity increases, and circulation and oxygen delivery improve. The body becomes more physically fit for the demands on it. As training progresses, the exercise stimulates only a mild stress response that quickly subsides without any serious consequences. Eventually, exercise ceases to be a significant stressor and will stay that way as long as the person stays adapted to the physical challenge

Infection is another example of a situation where the stress response is followed by a specific adaptation. An invasion by a previously unknown pathogenic microorganism is a serious stressor and prompts a stress response regardless of the nature of the pathogen. At the same time, the immune system quickly shuffles through its ranks and finds the most fitting "soldiers" to fight this particular invader. These weapons (such as antibody-producing cells) are perfected through several stages of biochemical transformation and multiplied into millions of copies until the pathogen is destroyed. The stress response subsides and the adaptation is complete.

The immune system remembers the pathogen and will be prepared for another invasion. What started as a general stress response ended as a long-term specific adaptation. This ability to learn from previous attacks is the basis for the use of vaccines.

There are situations in which the body fails to develop specific adaptation to a stressor, inevitably leading to a prolonged and damaging stress response. Some common examples of this are abusive relationships, unresolved grief, constant job pressure and sleep deprivation.

There's no doubt that the body's capacity for specific adaptation declines with age. However, as one gets older the stress response does not diminish. On the contrary, it becomes progressively more excessive. As we age, normal body chemistry is disturbed in such a way that the systems responsible for keeping the stress response in check become less effective. However, there is also another reason why older people have an excessive stress response. In the young, the stress response is comparatively brief, quickly followed by an efficient specific adaptation, keeping damage caused by stress to a minimum. In older individuals, specific adaptation is slow or sometimes impossible due to the less efficient functioning capacity of the body's systems. When the body cannot develop specific adaptation, its only recourse is to maintain the stress response as long as it can. This can lead to exhaustion and disease.

WHAT CAN BE DONE TO RESTORE OUR ADAPTIVE ABILITY TO YOUTHFUL LEVELS?

- **Measures aimed at slowing down the mechanisms of aging** (discussed throughout this book) can help to preserve your adaptive capacity by preserving the function of vital organs and tissues.
- **Adaptogens** This is a unique class of agents that provides two benefits. Adaptogens both optimize the stress response and improve the body's ability to adapt. This unique combination makes them an effective tool for life extension and disease prevention. Most adaptogens are nutrients or plants extracts and usually have no or few side effects. Chapter 28 is devoted to the benefits of adaptogens and their use.
- **Regular exposure to "good stress"** Regular exposure to moderate short-duration physical stressors, such as exercise or yoga, stimulates adaptive systems and keeps the body better prepared for serious stressors. A person conditioned by exercise or yoga tends to have a milder stress response and achieves a lasting adaptation to various physical and emotional stressors more quickly.

Another frequently overlooked feature of adaptation is that it makes better sense to maintain a state of adaptation rather than adapt all over again every time there is a need for it. In other words, it is better to stay in good shape than get yourself in shape once in a while. The rationale behind this is simple, with a strong heart, lungs, muscles and a well-balanced immune system, the body will usually adjust faster to adverse conditions without going through an intense stress response. However, when a person has to adapt each time from scratch, the body undergoes an intense stress response and suffers all the damage associated with it. The bottom line is: if you decide to engage in exercise or yoga, stick with it. Two to three times a week is more than sufficient - just keep it up.

Maintaining the state of adaptation (i.e. staying in shape) becomes even more important as we grow older to preserve tissues from stress-related damage. Also, the stress response is slower to react and even slower to shut down when the emergency is over.

Inhabitants of the Peruvian Andes are well adapted to their high altitude of 13,000 feet. They have more red blood cells, stronger heart and lungs and higher density of capillaries in their tissues. But if the elderly inhabitants move to sea level and return to the mountains in a few months, many would develop chronic altitude sickness. Their altitude sickness is a state of chronic stress caused by an inability to adapt.

A more familiar example of the inability to adapt resulting in the state of chronic stress is congestive heart failure, or the inability of the heart muscle to pump enough blood. This condition is very common among the elderly and is often precipitated by heart attack and hypertension.

Normally, when someone requires more blood flow than the heart is capable of providing, the heart muscle grows in size and gradually adapts to the increased demand. In heart failure, however, this adaptation doesn't occur and the body's only recourse is a perpetual stress response. In many patients, stress is so intense that people become severely underweight, and much of their lean tissue breaks down as a result of excess stress hormones.

One can reduce the risk of developing heart failure by improving the body's general adaptive capacity as well as taking preventative steps at the first signs of heart disease or malfunction. The adaptogens discussed in chapter 28 can help with general adaptation. Nutrients like coenzyme Q10 and L-acetyl-carnitine can boost energy production in the heart muscle and increase its functional capacity. This may help and prevent or in some cases, even reverse heart failure.

CHAPTER 15

STRESS AND AGE-RELATED DEGENERATIVE-DISEASES

Bad things happen to good people. However, the risks are not the same all the time. For example, the risks of illness or disease is far greater during or after a stressful experience. Traumatic experiences such as the loss of a loved one, being fired from your job or simply picking up stakes and moving your home can increase your risk of becoming ill. These may be as trivial as a cold or headache, but they can also be extremely seriously ailments like ulcers or a fatal heart attack. Stress also tends to worsen existing conditions.

Stress promotes disease because the body's stress response can have serious side effects. For instance, stress increases free radical damage, blood pressure and impairs immunity. In chapter13 we've discussed in great detail how stress accelerates the aging process by potentiating its key mechanisms. So it's not surprising that the progression of degenerative-diseases can be promoted by stress.

STRESS AND CARDIOVASCULAR DISEASE

Stress can inflict both direct and indirect damage to the heart. Stress dramatically increases the levels of "anxiety hormones" epinephrine (adrenaline) and norepinephrine (noradrenaline) which cause the heart muscle to contract more forcefully. In addition, these hormones increase blood pressure, placing an even greater strain on the heart.

Partial list of conditions whose onset or progression is strongly linked to stress

Angina
Asthma
Autoimmune diseases**
Cancer*
Cardiovascular disease*
Common cold
Crohn's Disease
Diabetes (Type II)*
Depression**
Fybromyalgia
Headaches
Hypertension*
Immune suppression*
Irritable bowel Syndrome
Multiple Sclerosis
Rheumatoid Arthritis
Ulcerative Colitis
Peptic ulcer

*** Age-related diseases**
****Possibly age-related diseases**

To work under these conditions, the heart must burn more fuel. This inevitably leads to the formation of large amounts of free radicals which can damage or destroy cells in the heart muscle. Unlike liver or skin cells, heart muscle cells are not easily replaced. The heart compensates for this loss mainly by enlarging and powering up the remaining cells. This works up to a point, after which clinical heart failure may occur.

In addition to avoiding stressful situations when possible, there are ways to protect the heart muscle from the ravages of stress. There is evidence that reasonably high doses of lipid-soluble antioxidants such as vitamin E or lipoic acid can significantly reduce damage to the heart. Research has found that adaptogens, the anti-stress agents discussed in chapter 28, also protect the heart muscle from stress.

The consequences of acute stress may interfere with the heart function by disrupting its normal rhythm. This effect is produced by the rapid release of large amounts of anxiety hormones during intense stress. Serious disturbances of heart rhythm can lead to profound disruption of the heart function and death. You can literally be scared to death, die in an outburst of anger or following some serious trauma. This isn't some second-rate B movie plot. It happens every day in real life.

Every year, over 400,000 people in the United States die suddenly. Presumably, the main cause is ventricular fibrillation, a severe disturbance of the heart rhythm in which the heart ventricles begin to flutter uncontrollably and are unable to contract in normal fashion. In a 1971 article published in the Annals of Internal Medicine, Dr. G. Engel analyzed 170 cases of sudden death. Most occurred shortly after a highly stressful event, such as a threat or loss of someone close, personal danger or even intense joy.

Here are some telling examples:

> A man of fifty-two had been in close contact with his physician during his wife's terminal lung cancer. He died suddenly of a massive myocardial infarction the day after his wife's funeral.
>
> A 40-year-old father slumped dead as he cushioned the head of his injured son lying on the street after a motorcycle accident.
>
> A middle-aged college president who prided himself on his support of black students died when a group of black students occupied the administration building.
>
> A seventy-five year-old man, who hit the twin double for $1,683 on a $2 bet, died at the pay window.

Of course, it is nearly impossible to avoid all severe stress completely. Nonetheless, the state of the body at the time of a stressful event may either predispose or protect a person from sudden death. For instance, the heart muscle's sensitivity to catecholamines is heightened by potassium and magnesium deficiency and reduced by high intake of these minerals. A high intake of potassium and magnesium, abundant in fruits and vegetables, is likely to reduce the risk of sudden death. The amino acid taurine is another nutrient that pacifies the heart and reduces the risk of sudden death from acute stress. In various studies, about 60% to 90% of sudden death victims had preexisting coronary heart disease. Rhythm disorders are known to be much more likely in the heart that does not receive enough oxygen because of partial blockage of coronary arteries by atherosclerotic plaques.

Atherosclerosis is another example in which stress contributes to heart disease. Stress hormones induce several metabolic shifts that promote atherosclerosis, including elevated blood sugar, insulin resistance and increased levels of free fatty acids. In addition, stress favors the development of hypertension which is a strong risk factor for atherosclerosis.

There are a number of studies linking behavior with the risk of cardiovascular disorders. Evidence indicates that individuals who exhibit Type A behavior pattern (TABP) tend to have a higher risk of heart disease. Dr. Ray Rosenman, an expert in the behavioral risk factors of heart disease, defined TABP as follows:

Individuals who are in a relatively chronic struggle to do and achieve more in less time, often in competition with others, exhibit the set of behavior known as the Type A behavior pattern. The TABP includes such behavioral dispositions as ambitiousness, aggressiveness,competitiveness, and impatience; specific behaviors such as alertness, muscle tenseness, rapid and emphatic speech patterns; and emotional reactions such as enhanced irritation and expressed signs of anger.

In psychological terms, hyperactivity (TABP behavior) is linked to stressors, when most events and situations are perceived (often subconsciously) as stressful. As a result, the body's stress response is on most of the time, contributing to the development of heart disease.

We should note here that TABP is not a personality characteristic, but largely a type of behavior that can be learned and unlearned given enough incentive.

In a competition-driven culture, society provides more than enough incentives to learn TABP behavior-rewarding achievement, excellence, winning, and relentless striving. The best incentive to modify TABP behavior is its potential for lowering the risk of heart disease. Unfortunately, it often takes a heart attack to provide sufficient motivation for a person to unlearn TABP.

Countless volumes have been written about behavior modification for the sake of one's health. The subject is far too vast to address in this book. We will only note that one of the key factors at the heart of TABP is the desire and effort to control as much of one's environment as possible. With much of our world beyond our control, this attitude would lead to frequent disappointments, frustrations, anger and a higher level of stress. We do not mean to say that one should completely relinquish control over one's life, to just relax and go with the flow, but as Dr. Sander Orent writes in "Stress and the Heart"; "What appears to be necessary for Type A's then, are an assessment of priorities, and an ability to sort relevant from irrelevant challenges. How important is it to become enraged during a traffic jam, or to endure the internal catecholamine storm [release of anxiety hormones] for the sake of job advancement, if the consequence could be coronary heart disease?"

Stress and hypertension

Hypertension is defined as arterial blood pressure at or above 140/90. While often asymptomatic, this silent killer can dramatically increase the risk of stroke, heart failure, kidney and eye disease. Excessive high blood pressure can cause damage by putting excessive strain on the entire cardiovascular system.

The causes of hypertension are complex and still not fully explored. Often, some combination of the following three factors are responsible: increased volume of blood, increased vascular resistance (the vessels are excessively constricted not allowing the blood to flow "easily") and increased cardiac output (the heart pumps with excessive force).

The level of stress can influence all three of these factors. Stress steroids may cause blood volume to increase by inducing retention of sodium and excretion of potassium by the kidneys. Anxiety hormones and the sympathetic nervous system make the heart work harder, causing blood vessels in most organs to constrict. The result is hypertension.

Elevated blood pressure during stress is just part of the problem. Evidence indicates that frequent stress can affect the control setting in the brain in such a way that blood pressure remains elevated when there is no stress. Most studies agree that people whose stress response is especially strong and easily triggered are at significantly greater risk of developing hypertension. The development of persistent hypertension is preceded by a period of so-called labile hypertension, when blood pressure elevations are episodic and occur mainly under stress. The greater and more frequent the stress, the higher the chance of labile hypertension progressing to chronic stress.

Epidemiological studies indicate that hypertension is much more prevalent in Western society and is often attributed to a diet low in potassium and magnesium and high in sodium and saturated fats. However, we believe that this is only a small part of a much bigger picture. Psychological stress which is endemic to Western culture should bear much of the blame.

Conventional treatment of hypertension relies on a variety of drugs that relax blood vessels, calm the heart or reduce blood volume and increase sodium excretion by the kidneys. Most of these drugs produce serious side effects.

It is particularly true in the case of hypertension that an ounce of prevention is worth a pound of cure. One simple measure you can take to prevent hypertension is a diet high in potassium and magnesium and low in sodium. In other words, eat plenty of fruits and vegetables and hide the salt shaker. Regular exercise and relaxation also help prevent hypertension. Adaptogens like Siberian Ginseng are also effective in preventing hypertension.

Keep in mind that serious hypertension is extremely dangerous and should not go untreated. Your physician can prescribe drugs that will help you keep this silent killer from claiming you as its next victim.

STRESS AND CANCER

Cancer is a complex disease. Many factors can contribute to its development including diet, exposure to carcinogens, aging, family history and one other potential suspect, stress.

The controversy over the role of stress in the development of cancer has been bandied about for several decades. Animal studies show that when stressed animals are exposed to carcinogens, their risk of developing tumors is greater. When cancer cells are injected into animals, those under stress show a faster progression of the disease.

Are these studies relevant to us? After all, methods employed to produce stress and cause tumors in laboratory animals are quite different from the typical events of our everyday lives. It's not impossible to study the effects of stress on cancer patients directly. In essence, researchers select a group of cancer patients and another group of cancer-free subjects. The groups are identically matched in age, sex and as many other variables as possible. Next, the researchers determine the number of individuals in each group under severe or prolonged stress within the test period. If the group with cancer had significantly (statistically) more stressful events in the past than the control group, this would suggest that stress may be one of the key causes of cancer.

Many such correctional studies have been done. The majority indicate that stress does contribute to the development of cancer. Especially pertinent is the current data on breast cancer, the leading type of malignancy in women. A Greek study of 1,088 patients found a very significant correlation between stress and breast cancer. Types of stressful events that correlate with cancer included the death of a loved one, negative behavior of a spouse, an unexpected change in life style, continual family conflicts, financial problems, unsatisfactory sex life, consultations with psychiatrists and allergies. Remarkably, the correlation between breast cancer and stress was stronger than with any other risk factor, including family history.

A British study conducted on 2,163 women also found a correlation between major stressful events and breast cancer. The link was especially strong in those women who were unable to express their emotions and obtain appropriate help and counseling. In a 1996 review of the literature on the subject, C.M. Bryla concludes that although the difficulty of measuring stress makes it hard to demonstrate a tangible relationship between stress and breast cancer, studies reveal that stress is related to breast cancer in various ways.

Assuming the relationship between stress and cancer is genuine, what could be its mechanisms? One possibility is that a flood of free radicals unleashed by stress may cause additional mutations in the genes and thus increase the risk of cancer. Another possibility is that cancer cells appear in the body quite often, yet the vast majority are defeated and destroyed by the immune system (mainly by natural killer and T-killer cells). Only occasionally does a cell escape the tight surveillance of the immune system and develop into a tumor. It is believed that spontaneous remissions (rare events when cancer completely regresses without treatment) are due to the "awakening" of the immune system to the presence of cancer.

Stress, however, can markedly suppress the activity of the immune system and presumably weaken the body's anti-cancer defenses. In animals and people under stress the activity of natural killer and T-killer cells is generally depressed.

According to recent research, one of the reasons for the limited effectiveness of conventional cancer-treatment methods (surgery, chemotherapy and radiation) is that they produce stress severe enough to dramatically suppress the immune system. This allows any surviving cancer cells in the body to grow and spread without hindrance. Many animal and some human studies showed that combining conventional cancer treatment with agents that mitigate the stress response (such as adaptogens) and/or stimulate the immune system which reduces the incidence of relapse.

In the previous section we've learned that heart disease is linked to type A behavior. More recently, scientists have attempted to define a another pattern of behavior associated with a higher risk of cancer. This cancer-prone behavior was named Type C and surprisingly, found in many ways to be the extreme opposite of Type A. Type C individuals are characterized by the denial of traumatic events, suppression of emotions, "pathological niceness," avoidance of conflicts, over-compliance and over-patience. Doctors in Germany, who reviewed the research on Type C behavior and cancer point out that this pattern often concealed behind a facade of pleasantness, appears to be effective as long as both environmental and psychological homeostasis is maintained. However, it usually collapses in the course of time under accumulated strains and stressors, especially those evoking feelings of depression and reactions of both helplessness and hopelessness. One of the most prominent features of this coping style is excessive denial, avoidance, suppression and repression of emotions. In fact, one's own basic needs appear to weaken the individual's natural resistance to carcinogenic influences.

Evidence indicates that the inadequate and repressive coping style found in Type C behavior is associated with a disproportionately prolonged stress response that leads to the suppression of many aspects of immunity, including anti-cancer defenses.

We also noted earlier that Type A behavior increases the risk of heart disease by excessively stimulating the stress response. If both Type A and Type C behavioral patterns affect health by amplifying the stress response, then why does one promote heart disease and the other cancer?

Apparently, Type A and C behavior engage the stress response in entirely different ways. In Type A individuals, the first fight or flight phase of the stress response is excessively intense, creating high levels of anxiety hormones, elevating blood pressure and placing an extra load on the heart and arteries. In Type C individuals, the fight or flight reaction is relatively weak, but the following phases of the stress response are excessively intense or prolonged due to poor coping ability. High levels of the stress steroids seen in these later phases suppress the immune system, and may impair anti-cancer immune defenses. Similarly to Type A, Type C is not considered a personality type, but rather a pattern of behavior that can be learned or unlearned. The steps towards overcoming Type C behavior involves allowing oneself to feel, communicate one's emotions to others, and to use counseling and support groups in times of crisis. One should keep in mind that Type A and Type C behavior are extremes of a very wide spectrum.

It's also important to note that by unlearning Type A behavior, one does not automatically become a Type C or vice versa. Healthwise, the ideal behavior is right in the middle of them.

Of course, significantly changing one's behavior is difficult for some and impossible for others. Not every environment is conducive to change and many truly stressful events cannot be easily avoided. Nonetheless, it still may be possible to reduce the negative impact of stress on the risk of cancer by mitigating the stress response and stimulating the immune systems with nutrients and dietary supplements.

Stress and diabetes

The American Diabetes Association estimates that diabetes results in 176,000 deaths each year, plus 54,000 amputations and 24,000 cases of blindness. While this disease may produce no symptoms, its complications include heart disease, stroke and nerve damage, kidney failure, and degeneration of the retina.

Diabetes is defined as a persistent elevation of blood glucose. According to the new guidelines of The American Diabetes Association released in 1997, a person is considered diabetic if their fasting blood glucose level was at or above 125 mg/dl on more than two occasions. The two types of diabetes are I and II. Type I insulin dependent diabetes (*DDM*), usually starts early in life, and is characterized by the almost complete inability of the body to produce insulin which is the hormone required by most cells to consume glucose. Type II, noninsulin dependent diabetes (*NIDDM*), tends to occur in midlife or old age. The body produces insulin but the cells do not respond to it.

Diabetes is a common disease affecting about 5% of the population with at least 90% of the cases being type II. In the elderly, the incidence of diabetes is over 20%. Furthermore, there is an even larger number who are prediabetic (also called carbohydrate/glucose intolerant or latent diabetic). In this subgroup, glucose levels are higher than desirable but fall somewhat short of the standard definition of diabetes. It is noteworthy that the national criteria for diabetes has been recently readjusted for lower levels of blood sugar. This would seem to indicate the above estimates of prevalence are probably too low.

No matter how it's calculated, diabetes is highly prevalent and its risk increases with age. Further, some degree of carbohydrate intolerance is so common that it is considered by some scientists to be a part of "normal" aging. According to Dr. Dilman, the preservation of carbohydrate tolerance should be one of the mainstays of an anti-aging strategy. Indeed, studies in rodents showed that improving carbohydrate tolerance extends life span. A variety of difficulties have so far prevented conducting similar studies in humans. It is remarkable, however, how many of the long-term complications of diabetes resemble some of the signs of premature aging.

Stress appears to be one of the risk factors in the development of prediabetes and type II diabetes. Others include ages over forty, obesity, lack of physical activity and possibly, chromium deficiency. Stress can also dramatically exacerbate existing diabetes.

Stress has a profound effect on the metabolism. It also has a profound effect on the body's ability to utilize glucose. As we have noted throughout this book, one of the principal biological purposes of the stress response is to provide extra fuel for heightened activity of the circulatory and nervous systems in an emergency. This is accomplished by increasing the levels of blood glucose; i.e., shifting the body chemistry closer to a diabetic state. It remains unclear whether stress can be the sole cause of diabetes. However, it just may be the final straw that tilts the body's homeostasis towards diabetes.

In previous chapters we've noted that the body's production of stress steroids increases with age. In other words, in terms of body chemistry, older people tend to live in a state of chronic stress. This may be one of the reasons why diabetes is an age-related disease.

CHAPTER 16

STRESS AND THE IMMUNE SYSTEM.

An immune system in good working order is essential for both short and long-term survival and longevity. It is the body's principal defense mechanism against infection and degenerative-diseases. It also plays a role in preventing some degenerative-diseases such as cancer and atherosclerosis.

As we age, the immune function declines, leaving us more vulnerable to infection and disease. Aside from aging itself and nutritional deficiencies, stress is perhaps the greatest threat to the body's immune system.

The young are resilient and often able to withstand a temporary impairment of their immune system. The elderly have fewer reserves and cannot afford to suffer a compromise in immunity. Furthermore, the elderly tend to be more vulnerable to the ravages of stress due to the overproduction of stress steroids. It is critical then to know how stress suppresses the immune system and what can be done to prevent or even reverse the damage.

The impact of stress on the immune system in animals was clearly demonstrated by Hans Selye in the Thirties. He found that animals subjected to stress had shrunken thymus glands and atrophied lymph nodes, which clearly indicated decreased activity of the immune system. Later, using more sophisticated methods, stress was shown to affect almost all aspects of the immunity.

Dissimilar stressors like loud noises, immersion in cold water or electric shock were found to impair immunity in laboratory animals. Purely psychological stressors can prove just as detrimental to the immune system as any physical stressor. Both social isolation and overcrowding impair immunity in mammals. Peer and maternal separation dramatically suppress immunity, especially in young animals. In one study, infant macaques separated from their mothers for two weeks were found to produce significantly fewer immune cells. Conversely, the reunion of the animals enhanced their immunity.

Numerous studies in rodents have demonstrated that stress accelerates the growth of tumors and promotes the spread of metastases as well as overall cancer mortality. Most researchers believe that these effects result from stress-induced immunosuppression, especially the impairment in the function of natural killer cells and T-lymphocytes.

It is not yet fully understood how stress suppresses the immune system. Scientists believe that stress steroids released by the adrenal glands are the main culprits: they suppress growth of immune cells and may even cause the self-destruction of others. Additional stress hormones join in and batter the immune system.

There can be no doubt that stress suppresses the immune system in laboratory animals and increases the likelihood of infection and cancer. But does this hold true for humans in the real life maze of stressful situations like divorce, marital problems, death of a family member, a change in social status or work pressures? Most doctors would agree that stressed-out people get sick more frequently. However, can clinicians corroborate this?

Human research on the subject is limited, but existing evidence indicates that the stresses of real life do indeed effect the immune system and increase susceptibility to disease.

A series of studies was conducted at Ohio State University on the effects of various real life stressors on the immune system. In one study, 50 first year medical students were evaluated during exam periods (high academic stress) and between them (low academic stress). Examinations were associated with higher levels of self-reported illness as well as impairment in several immune parameters, including T-killer cell killer function and interferon production.

In another study, researchers found that divorced or separated men suffered significantly more episodes of illness than married men.

Interestingly enough, the initiators of divorce showed less stress and better immunity during the first year of separation than noninitiators, but after a year, their situation reversed. The explanation suggested by the researchers was that initiators feel more in control and show less stress at first, but may partially lose their coping ability as the negative consequences of the separation became more obvious.

The first research linking specific infections to real life stressful events appeared in the early Fifties. In 1951 Dr. Tom Holmes published the results of a study demonstrating the relationship between real life situations, emotions and colds. Allegedly, the researcher's interest in stress-related illness was sparked by reports from friends and patients that they were most "apt" to catch a cold when their in-laws were visiting for prolonged periods. This eventually lead him to develop the famous Holmes-Rahe social readjustment scale (Chapter 3) linking the risk of illness and stressful events. In recent decades, various studies have demonstrated a connection between stress and such infections as tuberculosis, influenza, mononucleosis, ulcerative gingivitis and the onset and recurrence of genital herpes.

Why does stress have such a drastic effect on immunity? Why would the body have a physiological mechanism for suppressing its own defenses against infection? The stress response evolved from prehistoric times when our ancestors routinely faced imminent danger and severe hardships requiring a physiological mechanism aimed at activating the body's essential survival systems. Everything in life comes with a price tag but the body's resources are limited. When fuel and nutrients are shunted to the nervous and circulatory systems during stress, other systems such as the digestive and immune system are deprived of their resources. Their activity is suppressed to "balance the body's budget." Thus, the stress response increases the chances of overcoming the immediate threat as well as increasing the chances of long-term damage.

In both the primitive world and the animal kingdom this idea makes perfect evolutionary sense. If you are unable to survive the immediate danger in a struggle with a predator or you're unprepared for extreme heat or cold, it wouldn't matter much if your immune system is in tip-top shape. You'd likely be considered ancient history before the end of the day. On the other hand, you'd have a much better chance of surviving and producing offspring if you have two mechanisms to help you actually survive life threatening situations even though one mechanism - the stress response may impair the other (the immune system).

The only difference is that today's environment is significantly different than the one that shaped our environment. Truly life-threatening situations are rare for most of us, but psychological and social pressures abound. Unfortunately, we have not developed any significant adjustments to the stress response over the millennia, and our bodies react to a psychologically charged situation as if it were physically life threatening. The result is an excessive stress response leading to, among other things, impaired immunity.

Stress and autoimmune diseases

In essence, two things can go wrong with the immune system. First, it can simply become too weak, unable to mount a sufficient response to promptly and fully counter infections. Second, it can become "confused" and attack the body's own structures by mistake, causing autoimmune diseases such as rheumatoid arthritis and lupus. Aging tends to both weaken the immune system and increases the risk of autoimmune disorders. Stress, too, weakens the immune system and appears to have a profound, but if a less straightforward effect on autoimmune disorders.

The nature of the relationship between stress and autoimmune conditions depends largely on timing. In a patient with a full-blown disease, stress tends to somewhat reduce the severity of the autoimmune reaction and may actually temporarily alleviate some symptoms. This may be a result of the general immunosuppressive action of stress hormones. The onset or relapse of autoimmune disorders are often triggered by stressful events. The reasons for this are unclear, largely because the causes of autoimmune diseases in general are poorly understood. It is known that the majority of self-reacting T-cells are eliminated during their maturation in the thymus. What makes some self-reactive T-cells escape and attack the body's tissues is unknown. Stress is known to affect the thymus, causing it to shrink and lose some of its function. Scientists believe that stress may somehow disrupt the thymus' ability to weed out self-reactive T-cells, thus opening the gates for autoimmune disorders.

Most studies on stress and autoimmunity have involved rheumatoid arthritis, one of the most common autoimmune conditions, affecting about 1%-2% of the population. The immune system attacks cartilage, causing joint inflammation, pain, stiffness and sometimes deformity as well as disability. The onset of rheumatoid arthritis tends to follow either a single abrupt and highly stressful life event or a long-running series of unpleasant experiences. In the first category is the death of a loved one, divorce, termination of employment or abrupt loss of social status. The second includes long-term marital discord, increased work pressure or difficulties in child-rearing.

In one intriguing study, researchers studied pairs of identical female twins in which only one had rheumatoid arthritis. They found that the affected twin had experienced significantly more stressful life events prior to the onset of the disease, than the unaffected twin. The long-term course of rheumatoid arthritis also seems to be effected by stress. Several studies reported that the course and outcome of rheumatoid arthritis tends to be more benign in those patients who have a supportive social environment. Other autoimmune diseases whose onset was found to be affected by stress include: multiple sclerosis, autoimmune thyroid disorders and insulin-dependent diabetes.

CHAPTER 17

STRESS AND DEPRESSION

In Chapter 9, we discussed how depression can contribute to aging and conversely, how the risk of depression increases with age. Correcting depression is vital to life extension for two major reasons. First, depression intensifies several mechanisms of aging and second, it takes away the motivation and persistence required for the journey towards a longer and healthier life.

Stress is the most common cause of depression among humans and in animals. Animals get depressed just as humans do. In fact, stress is a standard tool used by researchers in animal studies on depression. When animals such as rats and mice are subjected to mild, unpredictable stress, they markedly reduce their intake of palatable food and sweet drinks. If animals are given an antidepressant, their intake usually returns to normal. This experimental model is often used to test the efficiency of new antidepressants before they are considered for human trials.

A wide variety of stressors can cause depression in humans. Job pressures, family problems, financial troubles, illness - almost any actual or perceived adversity can plunge a person into depression. It seems that depression develops when the body fails to limit its stress response after the stressor has been eliminated or neutralized. In a sense, depression is a self-perpetuating state of stress that can continue in the absence of any external stimuli.

Physiologically, depression resembles a state of chronic stress in several ways. The principal biochemical similarity between them is an increased level of stress steroids. This has a profound effect on the body, including suppression of the immune system, poor wound healing, increased breakdown of lean tissue, impaired glucose intolerance and loss of calcium from bones.

A type of depression with marked anxiety, often called anxiety-depression or anxious depression, has many similarities with the initial phase of the fight or flight stress response. In both cases, there is activation of the sympathetic nervous system and release of anxiety hormones (epinephrine and norepinephrine) from the adrenal medulla. These changes are largely responsible for many of the signs and symptoms seen in anxiety states and emotional stress, including rapid heartbeat, palpitations, muscular tension, tremors, sweating, nausea, "butterflies in the stomach", etc.

Another important link between stress and depression is *serotonin*, the neurotransmitter involved in many functions of the nervous system such as: appetite, mood and relaxation. Depression and anxiety are often associated with low levels of serotonin in the brain. The agents that raise serotonin levels, improve mood, reduce anxiety, facilitate positive emotions and produce general relaxation. In other words, they make you feel good and carefree. *Prozac*, arguably the most publicized antidepressant of all times, works by blocking the uptake of serotonin by the neurons, thereby increasing its level in the brain.

Serotonin plays a role in limiting the body's stress response. Initially, during stress, serotonin levels in the brain increase. This appears to be a part of the mechanism by which the body limits its stress response. Prolonged stress, however, appears to have the opposite effect. It depletes serotonin in several key areas of the brain, which can result in decreased stress resistance and depression.

Studies indicate that stress does not have to be severe or unusual to cause a long-term decrease in the serotonin level in the brain. This means that continuous stress, even if mild or moderate, increases your chances of developing depression.

What are the practical implications of the link between stress and depression? Clearly, a person can lower their risk of depression by avoiding, whenever possible, a stressful environment. Relieving depression improves stress resistance and prevents excessive response to stressors. Finally, nutrients or activities that improve stress resistance may ward off the onset of depression. In fact, some adaptogens (mostly natural agents that improve stress resistance and optimize stress response) have significant antidepressant action.

Physiological character	Depression	Stress
Blood levels of stress steroids	Increased	Increased
Blood levels of anxiety hormones (epinephrine and norepinephrine)	Often increased, especially in anxious depression	Increased
Activity of the sympathetic nervous system	Often increased, especially in anxious depression	Increased in the alarm phase of the stress response
Levels of serotonin in the brain	Decreased	Initial increase followed by a prolonged decrease if stress continues
Sensitivity of the hypothalamus to the feedback inhibition by stress steroids	Decreased	Decreased

Table 9. Similarities between the physiological characteristics of stress and depression.

CHAPTER 18

SEXUALITY AND STRESS

Most people know from experience that sexual desire and performance usually wane during times of severe or prolonged stress. This appears to be a natural part of the stress response. After all, the stress response itself shifts the organism's priorities toward overcoming immediate danger or obstacles. All other physiological functions, including sex, take a back seat to what the body perceives as a battle for immediate survival.

If stress is short-term the sex drive returns soon after the situation eases. One important exception, however, is when stress is caused by a man's need to perform. This may result in anxiety or even temporary impotence. Sometimes reassurance is a sufficient remedy. Relaxation techniques or mild relaxants can be of help. However, the best medicine for performance anxiety, is an understanding, caring partner. The truth is in a stable monogamous relationship performance anxiety is almost nonexistent.

Chronic stress may have a lasting effect on sexuality. In today's society, chronic stress is usually psychological and is often associated with depression and anxiety, which can result in a loss of sexual interest. Because older people are more prone to chronic stress and depression, what an elderly person may consider a "normal" loss of sexual desire, is often a result of latent depression or chronic stress.

Some of the hormonal changes induced by stress have a direct effect on sexual function. Psychological stress and some types of physical stress, such as anesthesia, major trauma or chronic illness, markedly depress testosterone levels in animals and in humans.

Testosterone levels may remain low long after the event. Stress also increases the levels of the hormone **prolactin** and high levels of it are believed to increase the risk of impotence.

Stress also contributes indirectly to the development of impotence by increasing the risk of degenerative-diseases and is also a contributing factor in the main cause of organic impotence.

Evidence indicates that adaptogens may be beneficial in restoring sex drive. A recent Korean study found that ginseng, a highly effective adaptogen, was effective in improving both sexual desire and potency.

Stress that may impair sexual function

- Depression, anxiety, subdued mood, lack of interest in sexual activity
- Constriction of peripheral blood vessels (especially during stress accompanied by marked anxiety), preventing sufficient blood flow to reproductive organs
- Decreased production of testosterone
- Increased production of prolactin
- Increased risk of degenerative-diseases, such as atherosclerosis, hypertension and diabetes that contribute to vascular and nerve damage implicated in physical impotence

CHAPTER 19

CELLULAR STRESS.

Despite what form a stressor may take, the body responds to it in exactly the same way. It initiates a "red flag" reaction called a stress response or general adaptation response. But what about individual cells? Do they also have a way of dealing with stressful situations?

Surprisingly, the answer is yes. Cells also have a form of stress response. The concept of homeostasis is also true on a cellular level. A detailed overview of cellular stress is of little importance to most people, but we'll briefly discuss two key strategies used by the cells to counteract various damaging impacts: the heat-shock response and the cellular adaptation response.

HEAT-SHOCK RESPONSE

No mammalian cell can withstand very high temperatures, which is just one of the reasons why our body temperature is so tightly maintained at about 98.6^{O}F (37 degrees Celsius). A small temperature increase (to 40°- 42°C) is not lethal because the cell has a so-called heat-shock response, quickly shutting down routine operations such as the production of "regular" proteins. Cells then begin to quickly produce large quantities of special proteins called heat-shock proteins which are normally present in the cells in small amounts. The heat-shock response is also evoked by many other damaging factors such as: radiation, hypoxia, toxins, heavy metals, viruses and ethanol. In other words, it represents a general emergency response to danger - a cellular "fight or flight" reaction.

How heat-shock proteins help the cell survive remained a mystery for some time. Amazingly, a diverse zoological menagerie consisting of bacteria, yeast, fruit flies and humans have very similar heat-shock proteins and responses. This sort of extreme conservatism in a protein throughout evolution is usually an indicator of its critical importance to the very basic mechanisms of life. Research in recent years has revealed that the principal function of many heat-shock proteins are to stabilize, preserve and facilitate the recovery of cellular structures, such as DNA and proteins. This can occur both during and after damaging situations. Normally, DNA and proteins are folded in a special manner so that they can execute their functions in the right way. High temperatures cause them to unfold, not only disturbing their normal routine, but also making them more vulnerable to damage by free radicals and aggressive chemicals. It was found that some heat-shock proteins attach themselves to the disrupted portions of cellular structures to protect them from further damage and facilitate the restoration of the normal structure.

Many recent studies indicate that the heat-shock response changes as we age. In particular, cells produce fewer heat-shock proteins in response to cellular damage. This may be partly responsible for the loss of stress resistance seen in aging. Indeed, if the system of emergency protection does not work properly, the resulting damage is far greater. Some scientists believe that many of the functional and structural changes seen in old cells result from a diminished or deranged heat-shock response.

The good news is that age-related impairment of the heat-shock response changes as we age. At least one well known anti-aging tool in animals, caloric restriction, was shown to significantly reduce the loss of the heat-shock response with age. Unfortunately, caloric restriction does not have the same benefits in humans and other primates. On the other hand, there is a vast amount of promising research on improving the heat-shock response in aging cells.

Also, scientists are searching for other alternatives to improve heat-shock response.

CELLULAR ADAPTATION RESPONSE

Our cells appear to have another emergency defense system in addition to the heat-shock response. It has been called by many names. However, for simplicity's sake, we call it the cellular adaptation response.

Like the body's stress response, the cellular adaptation response is evoked by a similar variety of influences like radiation, toxins, and carcinogens, to name but a few. The defense philosophy of the individual cell is pretty much the same as that of the organism at large. Whatever the source of the problem, standardized emergency methods are initiated.

Dr. I. N. Todorov, one of the authors of this book, studied cellular stress over a period of two decades and discovered a number of key mechanisms used by the cell to respond to stressors. He found that most types of cell damage disrupt the cell's ability to manufacture proteins. The key goal of the cellular adaptation response is to preserve or restore this ability. This is quite understandable considering that essentially all functions of the cell depend on proteins. Some proteins (enzymes) catalyze vital chemical reactions, while others transport fuel and building blocks inside the cell or remove waste. Still others protect, maintain and service DNA. One can say that proteins run the cell. Absolutely nothing vital to the organism can work without them. If protein synthesis is prohibited, the cell's delicate balance and all vital functions are compromised.

Here is a summary of the steps a cell takes to regain its balance in an adverse situation:

1. The cell pumps more energy into protein manufacture. This alone can be enough to neutralize mild damage.

2. If a damaging situation remains unresolved, the cell is forced to take more radical measures. Normally, some of the proteins manufactured by the cell are kept for internal needs. The rest, often a more sizeable portion, are exported outside the cell to fulfill the need of the organism at large. For instance, liver cells export albumin, the main protein of blood serum. Pancreatic cells produce digestive enzymes and B-lymphocytes produce antibodies and so forth. When these first line measures fail, the cell shuts down the production of export proteins and whatever else it may be producing for the sake of the organism at large and rechannels the freed materials and energy into making the protein needed for internal purposes. In a sense, the cells temporarily relinquish all their responsibilities to the body to concentrate all their resources on survival.
3. The final phase in the cell's response to a prolonged and severe cellular stress involves DNA replication and cell division. Normally, cells divide when the body needs to grow or regenerate. It is not quite clear why cell division becomes a defensive measure. One possibility is that it helps to restore the correct proportion of principal cellular ingredients, DNA and proteins.
4. If the damaging situation remains unresolved even after cell division, the entire cycle will repeat itself.

A cellular adaptation response evoked by various stressors has important implications on the aging process. Firstly, it speeds up the rate at which the cell burns fuel. Secondly, the cellular adaptation response causes cells to divide more often. But cell division in higher organisms has a limit (see Hayflick limit in chapter 2). Thus cellular stress pushes the cells ever closer to this limit.

FIGHTING CELLULAR STRESS

In many cases, general (all-body stress) and cellular stress occur simultaneously. On one hand, stress hormones released by the body during the stress response appear to precipitate a cellular adaptation response and heat shock response in some tissues. Conversely, severe cellular stress in some vital organs would normally evoke an "all-body" stress response. Therefore, reducing the all body stress-response usually diminishes cellular stress and vice versa.

A more specific way to reduce cellular stress in a particular organ suffering from damage or excessive work load is to introduce so-called organ specific cytoprotectors (i.e., protectors of the cells). For instance, silymarin found in plant milk thistle (*silybum marianum*), prevents liver damage and other problems.

Ginkosides, active substances in ginko biloba, have a particular affinity to nerve tissue and can protect the nervous system from the ravages of free radicals or shortages in the blood supply. Para-aminobenzoic acid (PABA) protects skin from sun damage by blocking UV rays. Prostaglandin E1 (PGE1) prevents damage to the GI-tract cells by non-steroidal anti-inflammatory drugs, acid and acute stress. Coenzyme Q10 and acety1-L-carnitine protect the heart by improving its ability to generate energy.

We still have much to learn about cellular stress. In the near future, it may be possible to develop effective methods of preventing or neutralizing cellular stress in a variety of tissues. One promising avenue, cellular stress training is similar to moderate exercise as a protector from all-body stress. Some substances or forces can mildly stimulate the cellular adaptation response, heat-shock response or DNA-repair system. A cell pretreated in such a way becomes much more resistant to damage because its defenses have been prepared for battle.

Some scientists believe that evoking a mild heat-shock response with a cautious short-term exposure to heat may help maintain cellular levels of heat shock-proteins and make cells more resistant to various types of damage. This means that hot baths or regular visits to the sauna may not only help you relax, but may actually contribute to your overall health and well-being. Keep in mind that with few possible exceptions, almost everything is good in moderation. Overuse of a sauna or other heat treatments might not be such a hot idea. People with heart disease and some other conditions should not expose themselves to intense heat, so before you venture into a sauna, consult your physician.

CHAPTER 20

STRESS LIMITING SYSTEMS

The sprinkler system in an office building goes off automatically when it senses a rise in temperature. Similarly, the body's stress response is triggered by potentially or actually harmful situations to ensure immediate survival under extreme conditions. Unfortunately, the stress response itself, especially if intense or prolonged, can also prove damaging to the body. It may exacerbate diseases or even shorten life span. To protect itself, an organism must have the capacity to limit the intensity and duration of the stress response whenever possible.

Fortunately, we have a built-in mechanism which shields the body from the consequences of its own stress response but some of these mechanisms deteriorate with age, leaving the body exposed to the damaging effects of an excessive stress response.

Some of the stress-limiting mechanisms act indirectly via the central nervous system by altering the brain messages regulating the stress response and some directly protect cells from the ravages of stress. Others appear to operate both directly and indirectly. To minimize stress-related damage, it is crucial to keep these mechanisms in good shape. Older or severely stressed individuals may benefit from enhancing their stress-limiting mechanism through specific nutrients, supplements and other methodology.

Antioxidants systems The stress response generates a barrage of free radicals which can severely damage body tissues. At the same time, the initial phases of stress are associated with the stimulation of antioxidant defenses. This apparently counteracts the increase in free radical formation and thereby limits the damage. Severe or prolonged stress, however, eventually depletes antioxidant resources, leading to extensive cell damage. Our antioxidant reserves dwindle as we age. Older people produce fewer free radical-scavenging enzymes; their production of melatonin, a potent antioxidant, is virtually nothing. In addition, their levels of glutathione, the principal intracellular water-soluble antioxidant, are often decreased. Supplementary antioxidants, such as vitamin E, cysteine, lipoic acid, flavonoids and others, may help preserve antioxidant reserves under stress and prevent or reduce stress related damage. Older people benefit the most from antioxidant defenses as they tend to suffer more free radical damage. Specific information about supplementing your diet with antioxidants is given in Chapter 21.

Growth hormone (GH) Both physical and psychological stress, especially if intense, causes the release of growth hormone by the pituitary gland. Many researchers believe that GH release during stress limits the severity of the stress response and prevents or reverses the damage. Several studies have demonstrated that GH mitigates and reverses stress-related immunosuppression. Conversely, animals who do not secrete GH fail to recover their immune function when the stressor is no longer present. Stress steroids cause the loss of lean tissue by stimulating the break-down of protein for fuel. GH acts in the opposite direction, limiting the loss of protein and facilitating the restoration of lean tissue. As discussed earlier, GH production declines with age, and so does resistance to stress. Growth hormone production can be increased by the use of nutrients that stimulate the release of GH by the pituitary (see Chapter 25). The option of GH injections exists, as well, however, these are extremely costly with the added risk of adverse side effects.

GABA and GHB GABA (gamma-aminobutiric acid or gamma-aminobutirate) is an inhibitory neurotransmitter that has multiple effects on the nervous system. It produces muscle relaxation, reduces blood pressure, relieves anxiety and at high concentrations induces sleep. Its release stimulated by psychological and pain-related stress helps to mitigate the stress response. The effects of GABA are difficult to study because it does not cross the blood-brain barrier, so oral or intravenous administration produces little or no effect. GHB (gamma-hydroxybutiric acid or gamma-hydroxybutirate) is both a precursor and a metabolite of GABA. The two compounds are structurally related. Unlike GABA, GHB readily crosses the blood-brain barrier and once in the brain is converted to GABA. In addition to its precursor role, GHB appears to have a direct inhibitory action unrelated to GABA receptors. The administration of GHB to animals was shown to reduce the intensity of the stress-response and prevent stress-related damage to various organs, particularly the heart and gastrointestinal tract. In stressed animals treated with GHB, the release of stress hormones was reduced, as was the formation of free radicals in the heart muscle. Both GABA and GHB are considered nutrients. GABA is sold over-the-counter in health food stores. However, GABA is a relatively weak stress-protector because of its poor ability to cross the blood brain barrier. GHB was sold freely prior to 1990, when the FDA argued that GHB had a high potential for toxicity and abuse and banned over-the-counter sales in the US. This contention remains controversial. High doses of GHB do induce deep sleep from which a person cannot be easily aroused. However, so can high doses of several readily available substances such as alcohol. Unlike these substances, GHB does not appear to have any significant long-term toxicity and does not produce addiction or significant tolerance. **Diazepam** (Valium) and other benzodiazepines, which are widely prescribed tranquilizers and anti-anxiety drugs, work by acting on GABA receptors, simulating the release of GABA in the brain. These drugs appear to have far higher potential for abuse and tolerance than GHB. The debate on of GHB continues and we may yet see its return to one of availability.

<u>Enkephalins and endorphins</u> Enkephalins and endorphins (also called endogenous opioids) are morphine-like substances produced by the body. Their best-known effect is to decrease the perception of

pain. Various types of stressors, such as surgery, trauma or examinations cause the release of endogenous opioids. In some people, they not only reduce pain but also create a state of euphoria. The infamous adrenaline rush craved by thrill seekers is produced in part by endogenous opioids. During stress, endorphins and enkephalins accumulate in the hypothalamus and adrenals and appear to have a role in curtailing stress response. Administration of opioids to animals prior to stress prevents stress-related damage to the heart as well as stress-induced increase in metastatic dissemination of cancer. The amino acid D-pheylalanine inhibits the degradation of enkephalins, raising their levels in the central nervous system. D-phenylalanine was shown to reduce pain perception in animals. Some, but not all human studies showed D-phenylalanine to relieve pain, the response rate ranging from 32% to 75%. D-phenylalanine may help mitigate the stress response by elevating the levels of endogenous opioids. D-phenylalanine is considered a nutrient and is available over the counter, usually sold in a mixture with a closely related compound L-phenylalanine. L-phenylalanine is the precursor in the synthesis of neurotransmitter dopamine and norepinephrine. DL-phenylalanine (the equal mixture of D- and L-pheylalanine) was proven to relieve depression, being at least as effective as the common antidepressant, imipramine, but with fewer adverse side effects.

<u>Melatonin</u> In a strict sense, melatonin is not part of the organism's stress-limiting mechanism because its production is not increased by stressors. However, the ability to produce melatonin appears important in maintaining the body's resistance to stress. Melatonin helps minimize stress-related damage by stimulating the immune system and has a general calming effect. Several animal studies have demonstrated that melatonin prevented or reduced stress-related immuno-suppression and gastric ulceration. Production of melatonin declines dramatically with age, almost vanishing by the age of sixty. This may contribute to the loss of stress-resistance.

Although the stress response limiting mechanisms of the body are quite effective, they can be overwhelmed by severe or prolonged stress. These mechanisms often kick in when the stress response has been excessively stimulated and some damage is already unavoidable. Furthermore, some of the stress-limiting mechanisms lose efficiency with age, particularly the ones involving growth hormone, melatonin and free radical-scavenging enzymes.

Some stress-limiting systems can be enhanced by nutrient supplements. Supplementary antioxidants can help prevent the overload of the body's free radical scavenging systems during stress. Growth hormone releasers can markedly boost GH production, even in advanced age. DL-phenylalanine may be especially effective in pain-related stress and also when stress is accompanied by depression. Melatonin may improve stress-resistance in older people whose own production of the hormone is very low. GHB, the nutrient currently banned by the FDA, is a potentially useful tool in the anti-stress arsenal. Finally, some adaptogens, although not a part of the physiological stress-limiting mechanisms, used cautiously and judiciously, were shown to enhance or complement natural systems of stress resistance. We will discuss the practical details in Part III.

PART III

CHAPTER 21

EAT LIKE THERE IS A TOMORROW

Today, over 80 million Americans are fighting the battle of the bulge. They eat too much and are overweight. In a sense, the same thing keeping them alive is also killing them. Overeating.

Most of these individuals eat like there is no tomorrow. Which, for some of them, could be a self-fulfilling prophecy.

There is little doubt that the single most potent method of life extension and disease prevention in rodents is severe caloric restriction. To give you a better understanding of the effect food has on life span, let's start with the evidence that already exists. For example, rats restricted to 60%-70% of the calories consumed by their "all you can eat" counterparts, live up to twice as long, remaining healthy and agile long after the fat rats were dead and buried.

Caloric restriction is a potent inhibitor of aging and disease for rodents. The best results were achieved when caloric restriction was initiated early in life, before sexual maturation. This delays the rats development and therefore slows the central aging clock, leading to a dramatic increase in life expectancy. When initiated after maturity, this method is far less effective, yet still produces substantial health benefits and increases life span.

So why aren't we all on low-calorie diets? We would not only live longer, but we would also save a small fortune on clothes.

Unfortunately, caloric restriction does not have the same benefits for primates. Early caloric restriction in primates leads to aberrations in the central nervous system and decreases life span. There are indications that mild to moderate caloric restrictions after full maturity might be beneficial, but the jury is still out.

A more practical way to arrive at optimal caloric intake is to determine ideal body weight and adjust consumption accordingly. Ironically, the evidence linking body weight to life span comes mainly from large insurance companies. Since their premiums are based in part on mortality tables, clients are weighed at the time the policy is issued. According to this data, the longest life span is linked to a body weight somewhat below average (called desirable, ideal or optimal weight).

One should be aware that there are several limitations to the current data on desirable body weight:

- The weight range is based only on the lowest mortality rate among insured persons, which may not adequately reflect the population at large.

Relative Weight	Men	Women
20% Underweight	105	110
10% Underweight	94	97
10% Overweight	111	107
20% Overweight	120	110
30% Overweight	135	125
40% Overweight	153	136
50% Overweight	177	149
60% Overweight	210	167

Table 10. Mortality ratios according to variations in weight. Adapted from: Build study 1979. Chicago, Society of Actuaries and Association of Life Insurance Medical Directors, 1979. The study measured the deviation from a set of average weights when mortality would be 100.

Height without shoes (ft, in)	MEN Weight without clothes (lb)			WOMEN Weight without clothes (lb)		
	Acceptable Average	Acceptable weight range	Obese	Acceptable Average	Acceptable weight range	Obese
4' 10"				102	92-119	143
4' 11"				104	94-122	146
5' 0"				107	96-125	150
5' 1"				110	99-128	154
5' 2"	123	112-141	169	113	102-131	152
5' 3"	127	115-144	173	116	195-134	161
5' 4"	130	118-148	178	120	108-138	166
5' 5"	133	121-152	182	123	111-142	170
5' 6"	136	124-156	187	128	114-146	175
5' 7"	140	128-161	193	132	118-150	180
5' 8"	145	132-166	199	136	122-154	185
5' 9"	149	136-170	204	140	126-158	190
5' 10"	153	140-174	209	144	130-163	196
5' 11"	158	144-179	215	148	134-168	202
6' 0"	162	148-184	221	152	138-173	208
6' 1"	166	152-189	227			
6' 2"	171	156-194	233			
6' 3"	176	160-199	239			
6' 4"	181	164-204	245			

Table 11. Body weight guidelines

- Smoking tends to increase mortality in addition to lowering body weight. Consequently, for healthy non-smokers, this may lead to overestimating the weight associated with the lowest mortality.
- In most cases, being at a desirable weight indicates an optimal body composition. However, there are exceptions; a person with more fat and less muscle than optimal may still fall within the optimal weight range. A person with a well-developed musculature, may have optimal body composition but exceed the desirable weight. The first individual is likely to achieve some health benefits from weight loss, but the latter would not, although optimal weight tables may indicate the opposite.

With these limitations in mind, desirable body weight is a reasonable goal for someone pursuing life extension. In fact, maintaining desirable weight and body composition, especially in mid-life or at advanced ages, may offer similar caloric benefits. In rodent experiments, the control animals are fed *ad libitum*. In other words, they have an unlimited supply of and access to food. Not surprisingly, the animals overeat and become obese. Overeating is a natural mechanism which evolved under conditions of scarce food supply. Wild animals sometimes go without food for prolonged periods. Those with extra fat have a better chance of surviving. In the wild, it is advantageous to consume as much as possible in anticipation of the times when food is scarce or unavailable. Since animals given unlimited food tend to overeat, the life span comparison in caloric restriction experiments is not between starving and "slim" (desirable weight) rodents but, rather, between obese and slim rodents. In this context, persons who stays at desirable body weight are similar to calorie restricted rodents. It's no big secret that maintaining a desirable body weight usually requires self-discipline.

At present, one of the most practical ways to determine proper caloric intake for most people is to first determine one's desirable (ideal) bodyweight. Then one should tailor their caloric intake based upon achieving or maintaining this predetermined bodyweight.

Desirable body weight should be considered in the same light as achieving optimal body composition. The currently recommended range recommended ratio of fat to muscle mass for men is 18% to 22% and for women 18%-32%. Most experts recommend an absolute minimum of 5% to 10% fat for men and 12% to 16% for women.

Some fat is necessary to protect vital organs, support normal nerve impulse conduction and fuel reserve. The amount of "indispensable" fat in a woman is greater because her system requires extra fuel for child bearing. Women whose fat stores drop below a certain level cease to have menstrual cycles.

There are several methods for determining body composition; some more sophisticated than others. Most nutritionists measure the thickness of skinfolds at different parts on the body to arrive at an estimate. When properly done, this method is adequate. Some health clubs and specialized obesity treatment centers also offer methods such as underwater weighing and bioelectrical impedance.

When matching your weight to a desirable range, you should know your frame type (small, medium or large). A person with a small frame whose weight is at the top of the desirable range could have excess fat relative to the muscle tissue. Your nutritionist can help you determine your body composition, muscle and frame size.

LOSING IT WITHOUT "LOSING IT"

While the controversy on the optimal energy intake rages on, there is little doubt that being significantly overweight increases the risk of death and diseases. So achieving the desirable weight is an important part of life extension. However, this is just one of many factors and should be viewed as such. Even if you fail to achieve optimal weight, do not disregard taking other steps towards life extension and health.

Sadly, the general trend in many developed nations is towards overweight. New 1998 weight guidelines released by The National Institutes of Health, placed 55% of all Americans in that category. The guidelines use **body mass index** (BMI) as an assessment tool. You can determine your BMI easily: multiply your weight in pounds by 703, divide the result by your height in inches and divide this result by your height in inches the second time. A BMI greater than 25 suggests you are overweight.

The are no clear reasons for more than half of us being overweight. At the turn of the century, 90% of the workforce was engaged in agriculture or industry. This trend has shifted and now 90% of us work in offices doing less physically demanding work. Maybe it's the abundance of food, lack of exercise or the ubiquity of television. In any case, there is an enormous demand for weight loss treatments and products. Unfortunately, many people attempt a weight loss program using weight loss methods that are unhealthy and potentially dangerous.

Recently, the most dramatic example of a popular but damaging weight loss treatment was phen-fen, a combination of the prescription drugs phentermine and fenfluramine. Phen-fen was taken off the market by the FDA after it caused several deaths. Phen-fen is potentially life-threatening to the heart valves in up to 1/3 of its long-term users. Other drugs may be less deadly, but still produce a variety of side effects. Another popular weight loss drug is amphetamines which may also cause nausea, vomiting, cramps, dry mouth and anxiety. Amphetamines produce short-term weight loss by suppressing appetite. In most cases, however, the appetite returns to normal within a week or two despite continued use. Furthermore, after amphetamine usage has been discontinued, the appetite rebounds, leading to weight gain rather than loss.

Another common, unhealthy tactic in weight loss is impulsive dieting. A person goes on a very low-calorie diet, often inspired by a commercial weight loss organization or friend. Such diets are often deficient in multiple essential nutrients and may cause numerous adverse side effects, including headaches, nausea, and dizziness and in rare cases, even death. Furthermore, very low-calorie diets tend to cause weight gain in the long-term through a process called weight cycling. When energy consumption drops too far below expenditure, the body slows its metabolism to conserve energy. Once previous eating habits are resumed, the metabolic rate may remain a little below its pre-diet rate. Therefore, the dieter not only returns to his previous weight, but often exceeds it. Each diet cycle can lead to additional weight increase.

The two main types of body fat are central and peripheral. Central, or abdominal fat, located at the torso around the waist, has been linked to a number of diseases, including atherosclerosis, hypertension, and type II diabetes. Metabolic shifts associated with abdominal obesity include glucose intolerance, insulin excess and elevated blood lipids, all of which contribute to accelerated aging and development of degenerative-diseases. Peripheral fat, on the other hand, seems to carry much fewer health risks. A person oriented towards living a long and healthy life should be concerned with avoiding abdominal obesity. A simple and useful indicator of abdominal obesity is the waist-to-hip ratio. To arrive at your waist-to-hip ratio, divide the number of inches in your waistline by a number of inches around the hips. Waist-to-hip ratio of 0.8 + for women and of 0.95 + for men is associated with increased risk of obesity-related health conditions.

PRINCIPLES OF HEALTHY WEIGHT LOSS

1. Slowly but surely Weight loss should not be too rapid. It is not a race. If it is, chances are the dieter will begin weight-cycling and end up heavier than before. Besides, a desperate assault on one's weight can result in long-term health hazards. A pound of fat tissue stores about 3500 calories. Taking 500 calories out of your daily diet will result in losing about one pound per week. This pace can be sustained without slowing the metabolism and without creating uncontrollable food cravings. Negative energy balance can be created by any combination of eating less and expending more energy through exercise or physical work. Whatever regimen you choose, it's important to be consistent and patient.

2. Reason and moderation Simple, reasonable, consistent measures

can take you a long way toward reaching your ideal weight. Several studies demonstrated the link between excessive TV watching and obesity. Watching TV requires very little energy, expenditure is low, and viewers tend to have high calorie snacks. Cut your TV time as much as you can. Even better, replace it with exercise or outdoor activities.

More often than not, people eat more than they need to feel satiated. This is especially true when food is gobbled, instead of consumed at a more reasonable pace. Two things inhibit the hunger center in the brain, the fullness of the stomach, and levels of glucose and fatty acids in the blood stream. Rapidly eaten food isn't given time to be absorbed and tell your brain that your hunger is satisfied. As a result, you consume more than you need. Your mother knew what she was talking about. Eat slowly, chew thoroughly, and take time to enjoy your food. This way you will not only consume less food, but absorb more vitamins and minerals. If during a meal, you find that you are no longer hungry but you still have food on your plate - stop. Don't eat late at night, especially within 2-3 hours of going to bed. Energy expenditure during sleep is low, so much of a late-night snack is stored as fat. Make dinner the smallest, not the largest meal of the day. You need sizable meals for energy before your main daily activities, not after them.

3. **Dietary changes** Make reasonable changes in what you eat. You don't have to become a vegetarian or switch to a limited set of designated foods.

First, try reducing fat intake - especially saturated fat. Fat supplies 9 calories per gram. Protein and carbohydrates supply only 4 grams. Most Americans derive about 40% - 50% of their calories from fat. Limiting fat is the most effective way to cut calories. Most experts believe that fat should provide less than 30% of a person's total daily calories, and saturated fat, less than 10%. Strange as it sounds, there is some evidence that calories from fat are more "fattening" than calories from proteins and carbohydrates. In other words, among diets with the same amount of calories per day, those with higher fat content tend to be more fattening. In other words, you are what you eat.

The reason for that may have to do with how the body stores energy. Fat tissue is used as the body's primary long-term energy storage. Some food energy is expended on body functions. Most of the remainder, if any, is converted into fat for long-term storage. Converting dietary fat into body fat is an energy-efficient process because it's just replacing stored body fat. On the other hand, converting dietary carbohydrates into fat takes up a lot of energy, leaving less for storage. Thus when it comes to excess energy, fat calories are more "fattening" than calories from carbohydrates.

It's quite healthy to keep your carbohydrate intake at 55% - 70% of your total energy. Most of that should come from the complex carbohydrates found in grains, beans, and vegetables. A diet high in complex carbohydrates is beneficial for weight loss in several ways. First, carbohydrates are less easily converted to fatty tissue than fats. Second, carbohydrates stimulate the brain release of the neurotransmitter serotonin, a factor in inducing satiety. Third, complex carbohydrates tend to improve glycemic response to food and reduce insulin excess, one factor in obesity.

Avoid simple sugars whenever possible. Simple sugars are rapidly absorbed and cause blood glucose to spike. This results in insulin excess and sometimes reactive hypoglycemia.

Increase your fiber intake to at least 25 to 35 gms per day. Fiber provides a number of benefits for both weight loss and general health. It is best to increase your fiber intake by consuming high fiber foods, such as whole grains, vegetables, fruits and beans; fiber supplements may cause bowel obstruction and generally should be avoided. Increase your intake of fiber gradually to allow your system to adjust. This will minimize possible side effects of gas, bloating or diarrhea.

Non-vegetable protein preferably should be derived from chicken, turkey and fish. These sources are generally lower in fat, particularly saturated fat. Soy is an excellent substitute for animal protein, with not only a high biological value, but it has also has been shown to decrease cholesterol and LDL.

<u>Exercise</u> It may be difficult to decrease caloric intake by 500 calories a day. The alternative is to burn 500 calories a day through exer-

cise. Unfortunately, this can be quite a feat. You would need to jog for 45 minutes, play tennis for an hour, or walk for an hour and fifteen minutes. For most people, the best approach is to decrease intake by 250 calories a day and do 30 minutes of aerobic exercise four times a week – both realistic goals. You don't need to overstrain. Exercise at 50% - 60% of maximal intensity, such as a brisk walk, should be adequate.

Mind over matter Being overweight often has several physiological and psychological factors. Physiological factors are usually more obvious and can be approached directly. Psychological factors are often hidden, and can range anywhere between suppressed emotional conflicts to low self-esteem and even loneliness. Dealing with deep-seated psychological problems usually requires personalized professional counseling. On the other hand, there are a number of simple steps you can take to change the way you relate to and interact with food.

Eliminate or avoid inappropriate eating stimuli. Don't shop when you 're hungry. Don't keep high-calorie convenience foods at home. Let other family members choose, buy and store their own sweets. Prepare snacks at home and carry them to avoid vending machines and convenience stores. When at home, eat only in one place and in one room. Make small portions look large (e.g. spread food out). Avoid waiting until you are starving (e.g., don't skip meals, don't eat too small meals).

Reinforce good food choices and behavior. Prepare appropriate foods attractively. Learn appropriate portion sizes and prepare only one portion at a time. Eat slowly, chew thoroughly, and pause several times during the meal. Enjoy eating for itself. Don't watch TV or read while eating. Whenever possible, eat your meals with other health conscious people. Exercise in a group of active, upbeat people. If possible, chose "high-fun" sports like as tennis, racquetball or basketball.

GLYCEMIC EFFECT OF FOOD

As we eat, enzymes in the gastrointestinal tract break food down into small molecules, such as simple sugars, amino acids and peptides. Many foods - from ice cream to popcorn - contain glucose or other carbohydrates that can be converted to glucose in the body. Usually, glucose is in the form of starch, a branched polymer made up of many molecules. Sucrose is a sugar consisting of one glucose and one fructose molecule. As food is digested, its glucose is released and absorbed into the bloodstream, causing the blood's glucose level to rise. How dramatic such a rise would be is depends on several factors: (1) how much glucose a meal contains; (2) the form of the glucose (e.g. starch or sugar); (3) the presence of other food ingredients (such as fiber, that affect the rate glucose absorption).

In terms of life extension and disease prevention, one should avoid dramatic rises in blood glucose. High blood glucose causes damage via several mechanisms. It accelerates glycation and cross-linking of vital cellular structures. It causes insulin excess, a factor in most degenerative-diseases and it also may increase free radical formation. Agents that lower blood glucose and reduce insulin excess were shown to increase life span in rodents.

The ability of foods to raise blood glucose varies considerably. Nutritionists rate the glucose-elevating effects of foods with the *glycemic index*. The higher the rise of blood glucose after ingesting a certain food, the higher its glycemic index. For pure glucose (white bread), the glycemic index is set at 100.

Generally, given nutritionally-equivalent choices, you should lean toward foods with a lower glycemic index. Most vegetables, except for carrots, beets, and potatoes, have a low glycemic index. Fruits have a relatively low index because their sugars are mostly fructose, a form of sugar which converts to glucose relatively slowly. High-fiber foods generally have a low glycemic index because fiber slows down both the digestion and absorption of nutrients. Among common foods, the ones with the highest glycemic index are processed foods,

Food	Mean
Breads	
Rye (crispbread)	95
Rye (wholemeal)	89
Rye (whole grain, i.e. pumpernickel)	68
Wheat (white)	100
Wheat (wholemeal)	100
Pasta	
Macaroni (white, boiled 5 min)	64
Spaghetti (brown, boiled15 min)	61
Spaghetti (white, boiled 15 min)	67
Star pasta (white, boiled 15 min)	54
Cereal grains	
Barley (pearled)	36
Buckwheat	78
Bulgar	65
Millet	103
Rice (brown)	81
Rice (instant, boiled 1 min)	65
Rice (polished, boiled 5 min)	58
Rice (polished, boiled 10-25 min)	81
Rice (parboiled, boiled 5 min)	54
Cereal grains (cont'd)	
Rice (parboiled, boiled 15 min)	68
Rye kernels	47
Sweet corn	80
Wheat kernels	63
Breakfast cereals	
"All bran"	74
Cornflakes	121
Muesli	96
Porridge oats	89
Puffed rice	132
Puffed wheat	110
Shredded wheat	97
"Weetabix"	109
Cookies	
Oatmeal	78
"Rich tea"	80
Plain crackers (water biscuits)	100
Shortbread cookies	88
Root Vegetables	
Potato (instant)	120
Potato (mashed)	98
Potato (new/white boiled)	80
Potato (Russet, baked)	116
Potato (sweet)	70
Yam	74

FOOD	MEAN	FOOD	MEAN
Legumes		**Sugars**	
Baked beans (canned)	70	Fructose	26
Bengal gram dal	12	Glucose	138
Butter beans	46	Honey	126
Chick peas (dried)	47	Lactose	57
Chick peas (canned)	60	Maltose	152
Green peas (canned)	50	Sucrose	83
Green peas (dried)	65		
Garden peas (frozen)	65	**Dairy products**	
Haricot beans (white, dried)	54	Custard	59
Kidney beans (dried)	43	Ice cream	69
Kidney beans (canned)	74	Skim milk	46
Lentils (green, dried)	36	Whole milk	44
Lentils (green, canned)	74	Yogurt	52
Lentils (red, dried)	38		
Pinto beans (dried)	60		
Pinto beans (canned)	64		
Peanuts	15	**Snack foods**	
Soya beans (dried)	20		
Soya beans (canned)	22	Corn chips	99
		Potato chips	77
Fruit			
Apple	52		
Apple juice	45		
Banana	84		
Orange	59		
Orange juice	71		
Raisins	93		

Gycemic index values are adjusted so that the index of white bread is 100. Glycemic index is defined as the blood glucose response to a food portion containing 50gm of available carbohydrates expressed as a percentage of the response to the same amount of carbohydrate from a standard form. In this case, white bread. (From Wolever, T.M.S World Rev. Nutr. Diet., 62:120-185,1990.)

low fiber starches, (such as puffed rice, corn flakes, instant potatoes, wheat bread), and simple sugars. Do not avoid these foods completely, but consume them in moderation. The glucose-elevating effect of foods with a high glycemic index is usually reduced when they are eaten together with low glycemic, high-fiber foods. A sweet dessert has less glycemic effect when eaten after a low glycemic meal, such as chicken with vegetables or pasta.

Balancing your diet

Everybody knows they should be eating the right foods, yet few actually do. By balanced diet nutritionists usually imply a diet that contains all the essential nutrients within an optimal range. This range is selected to prevent protein malnutrition and vitamin or mineral deficiencies. A balanced diet may be necessary, but is not sufficient by itself for a comprehensive life extension program. Clearly, malnutrition must be avoided, but to beat nature and derive the benefits of long life one may need some nutrients in greater amounts than is found in the typical well balanced diet. Figuratively speaking, a balanced diet is one brick in the foundation on which a life extension program is built.

The simplest and probably most feasible way people can adhere to a balanced diet is to follow the recommendations of the Daily Food Guide developed by the US Department of Agriculture. Adults are advised to consume daily:

- 6 to 11 servings of breads and cereals
- 3 to 5 servings of vegetables
- 2 to 3 servings of fruits
- 2 to three servings of meat and meat alternatives (fish, poultry, eggs, dry beans, nuts)
- 2 servings of milk and milk products

The three major components of foods, or **macronutrients** are proteins, carbohydrates and fats. Current guidelines on the consumption of macronutrients are:

- 10% - 20% of total daily calories are to be derived from protein
- 55% - 70% of calories from carbohydrate
- less than 30% of calories from fat; saturated fat should account fo less than 10% of calories

Keep in mind that each gram of protein, is about 4 calories, carbohydrates, 4 calories, and fat, 9 calories. Carbohydrate calories should come mainly from complex carbohydrates found in breads, cereals and potatoes. The amount of protein required is based on body weight rather than total calories consumed. Recommended daily allowances of protein for adults is 0.8g per kilogram (2.2 pounds) of body weight. Lesser amounts may lead to protein malnutrition which is characterized by depressed immunity, edema and poor wound healing. While protein deficiency is common in the developing nations, more socialized cultures usually consume amounts far above the RDA. Excess protein is burned as fuel and remaining nitrogenous waste is converted by the liver into urea to be excreted by the kidneys. A significant excess of protein places some undue stress on these organs and should be avoided, especially in individuals at risk of kidney and liver disease. Diabetes is the most common risk factor of kidney disease. Hepatitis and excessive alcohol consumption increase the risk of liver damage.

Recent evidence indicates that amounts of protein moderately above the RDA may stimulate growth hormone release when used in conjunction with exercise. Arginine, lysine and glutamine, the GH-releasing amino acids contained in protein, are believed to be responsible for this effect. People who wish to enhance the release of GH in their bodies may benefit from deriving about 25% of their daily intake of calories from protein. This should only take place when done in conjunction with significant physical activity (see Chapter 25). Fish, turkey and chicken are preferred sources of non-vegetable protein.

Soybeans appear to be the best plant source of protein because it lowers cholesterol and LDL. A significant cholesterol-lowering effect requires substituting at least 25 grams a day of soy protein for an equivalent amount of animal protein.

Excessive consumption of fat is discouraged because diets high in fat are usually high in calories and promote weight gain. In addition, some types of fat are associated with increased risk of certain diseases. In particular, excessive intake of saturated fat increases the risk of atherosclerosis, colon cancer and hypertension. An excessive intake of over fried polyunsaturated fat also appears to increase the risk of various cancers, possibly due to increased free-radical damage to DNA.

Extremely low fat intake can also have negative consequences. The human body can synthesize most, but not all the fatty acid it requires. The exceptions are linoleic and linolenic fatty acids often, called essential fatty acids (EFA). An EFA deficiency is associated with skin, kidney and liver disorders. EFA deficiency was thought not to occur in healthy populations. However, persons on a long-term, very low fat diet may develop marginal EFA deficiency. A reasonably low fat intake - as little as 10% of total calories, is sufficient enough to prevent EPA deficiency.

Saturated fat is the type most detrimental to health. It should be reduced to below 10% of total calories. The main sources of saturated fat are animals, such as beef, pork, poultry; dairy products and eggs. Choose skinless chicken or turkey over red meat. Use low-fat dairy products. Eggs are valuable for high quality protein, but should be used in moderation, no more than 3-4 a week.

Monounsaturated and polyunsaturated fat improves lipid profile, lowering cholesterol, LDL and triglycerides, and raising HDL. Keep in mind, however, that merely replacing saturated fat with mono and polyunsaturated fat won't help much if you are consuming excess calories. The richest sources of monounsaturated fats are olive and canola oil, and those of polyunsaturated fat are corn, sunflower and soybean oil. If you use commercial products with much unsaturated fat, you can take vitamin E supplement to minimize free radical damage.

Some commercial products, such as margarine or vegetable shortenings contain partly hydrogenated oil. Hydrogenation is the chemical process in which some of the double bonds present in polyunsaturated fat react with hydrogen. As a result, fat becomes more saturated and less fluid. In particular, hydrogenation turns some of the polyunsaturated fat into monounsaturated fat. There is one catch, however, there are two types of monounsaturated fatty acids - *cis* and *trans*. Natural sources have only the *cis* variety which is beneficial for lipid profile. Chemical hydrogenation, however, yields both *trans* and *cis* unsaturated fat (usually more *trans* than *cis*). The effect of *trans* monounsaturated fat on lipid profile is at least as bad as that of saturated fat. In that light, substituting margarine for butter makes a much smaller difference than one might think.

Fish oil is a rich source of a special type of unsaturated fat, omega-3 fatty acids, particularly eicosapentaenoic acid (EPA) and decosahexaenoic acid (DHA). Omega-3 fatty acid became known when researchers discovered a very low incidence of atherosclerosis and heart disease in the Inuit people of Alaska and Greenland, despite high-calorie, high fat and high cholesterol diet. Analysis of the foods in their diet, mainly fish and sea animals, showed high content of omega-3 fatty acids. How and why fish oil prevents heart disease appears to be complex and includes antithrombotic action (blood thinning) and modulation of immune responses. Other research into the effects of omega-3 fatty acids found that they may inhibit the development of some cancers. The best way to incorporate omega-3 fatty acids in your diet is to include two to four fish meals per week.

Fiber

Over the past few decades, researchers have elevated fiber from a practically useless non-nutrient filler to an important food constituent conducive to health and longevity. Chemically, fiber is a diverse group of plant polymers based on polysaccharide chains. In contrast to starch, which is another type of polysaccharide, fiber cannot be digested by humans. Instead, it passes through the gastrointestinal tract fully or partially intact. Large amounts of fiber in the diet make stools soft and bulky.

Fiber entered into the spotlight when physicians working in Africa noted a very low incidence of such typical "Western" conditions as heart disease, diabetes, obesity, colon cancer, diverticulosis and hemorrhoids. They also noticed that the local population consumed a very high fiber diet - their stool volume was several times greater than that of people in the West. The role of fiber in preventing diseases and obesity was hypothesized, spawning abundant research on the subject. It was found that fiber indeed provides a number of health benefits and may also retard some mechanisms of aging, mainly by improving glucose tolerance and reducing insulin excess.

There are two major classes of fiber: water-soluble (gums, pectins, some hemicelluloses and mucilages); and water-insoluble (cellulose, some hemiselluloses and lignins). Water-soluble fiber prevails in fruits, oats, barley, and legumes. Water-insoluble fiber is generally found in larger concentrations in vegetables, wheat and cereals. The physiological effects of the two types of fiber are somewhat different, but both provide important health benefits.

Water-soluble fibers	Water-insoluble fibers
• Delay transit of food through gastrointestinal tract, especially in its upper portion • Lower blood cholesterol levels • Slow starch breakdown and delay absorption of glucose in the bloodstream	• Accelerate food transit in lower gastrointestinal tract • Increase stool weight and volume • Slow starch breakdown and delay absorption of glucose in the bloodstream • Are fermented by microorganisms to yield short-chain fatty acids beneficial to the colon cells

Table 12. Physiological effects of fiber

BENEFITS OF FIBER

Studies indicate that a full spectrum of beneficial effects are derived from a high fiber diet that includes a variety of fiber from different sources: fruits, vegetables, unrefined cereals, and legumes. Taking a supplement with a single type of fiber is a less than optimal shortcut.

Improved glycemic response, and reduced insulin release Glycemic response to food is the extent to which blood glucose rises after a meal. Soluble fiber slows the passage of food through the upper portion of the GI-tract and also prevents the small intestine from absorbing nutrients too quickly. The net effect is a slower and smaller rise of blood glucose after a meal and a correspondingly lesser release of insulin. In our view, this ability of fiber to reduce glucose levels and insulin excess is its single most important health benefit. As we discussed earlier, high blood glucose and insulin excess contribute to the aging process and are major factors in the development of several degenerative-diseases, including atherosclerosis, hypertension and diabetes. Drugs that reduce blood glucose levels and insulin excess extend life span in animals. A high fiber diet may be able to do the same, with fewer side effects.

Colon cancer prevention Epidemiological studies show that populations consuming high-fiber diets have low incidence of colon cancer. Fiber may prevent colon cancer by binding and quickly removing carcinogens from the colon.

Lowering cholesterol Soluble fiber lowers cholesterol levels by binding bile. The role of bile, whose main components are bile acids, is to aid in the absorption of lipids (fats and cholesterol). Bile acids are synthesized by the liver from cholesterol. When food enters the small intestine, bile is released through a duct opening in the duodenum. Most of the bile is later re-absorbed in the lower portion of the small intestine. Soluble fiber in foods such as oats, barley and legumes bind bile acids and prevent their recycling.

Losing weight High fiber foods generally contain fewer calories and fat per gram. Also, fiber reduces the excess of insulin, the hormone that tells the body to store nutrients and gain weight. The balancing effect of fiber on blood glucose also prevents hypoglycemia which can cause intense hunger. Switching gradually to a high-fiber diet may be the single most important step one can take towards losing weight.

Other benefits Fiber helps prevent such generally benign but bothersome intestinal problems as hemorrhoids, constipation and diverticulosis. It also helps maintain normal intestinal bacterial flora and a healthy colon lining.

Possible side effects of high fiber consumption

The possible side effects of a high fiber diet are usually minor and easily manageable. When a person switches abruptly to a high fiber diet, they may experience abdominal discomfort and excess gas, so to avoid this, the transition should be gradual.

Fiber supplements (not high fiber foods) may create an intestinal obstruction, a serious problem sometimes requiring surgery. If you choose to take fiber supplements, use them in powder form and take them with a lot of fluids.

How much fiber do we need?

Expert opinions vary in their recommendations for fiber intake. Most sources recommend an intake of 20-35 grams per day, which is two to three times higher than the average American consumes. Increase your fiber gradually, over several weeks, allowing your GI tract to adapt. Drink plenty of fluids to help soften the fiber and allow a smooth transit. Try to get fiber from various sources: fruits, vegetables, whole grain cereals, legumes. Adhering to USDA Food Guide Recommendations (see chart on page 179) that include 2-3 serving of fruit, 3-5 servings of vegetables and 6-11 servings of breads and cereals a day, will easily provide the recommended fiber intake.

CHAPTER 22

FREE RADICALS -THE ENEMY WITHIN.

Free radical damage is one of the greatest contributors to the aging process. As we described earlier, free radicals are indiscriminately reactive chemicals that can damage any structure in the cell.

Although sunlight and radiation can cause free radicals, the most common source is the normal burning of fuel that occurs in every cell, every minute, every day of our lives. Generally, the more free radicals an organism produces, the shorter its life span.

Because they burn fuel at a very high rate, the brain and the heart are the two organs most susceptible to free radical damage.

In addition to contributing to the aging process, free radicals are one of the major culprits in the pathogenesis of many diseases. Free radicals cause the oxidation of lipids in LDL making them adhere to the arterial wall and promote atherosclerosis. Free radicals also damage brain cells in Alzheimer's disease. Inflammation in rheumatoid arthritis is largely a result of the release of free radicals by the immune system cells. Excess free radicals also increase the risk of cancer.

As free radicals are an inevitable by-product of cellular respiration, they cannot be entirely eliminated. However, the amount formed in the cells can be reduced. A number of things can be done toward reaching this goal.

Eliminating excess calories The amount of free radicals in our bodies are directly proportional to the amount of calories we burn. When cells burn a lot of fuel, they also produce a lot of "molecular soot," a.k.a. free radicals. In rodents, restricting the amount of calories by 30% - 40% increases life span up to two-fold. Eliminating excess calories and striving for optimal weight will reduce your exposure to free radicals.

Antioxidants Antioxidants are substances that neutralize free radicals rendering them harmless. Dr. Denham Harman, a pioneer in antioxidant research, found that mice on a diet containing 0.5-1% antioxidants had a 30% - 45% increase in life span. A number of nutrients, some of which are essential for survival, act as antioxidants. Various fruits, vegetables and plants are the most abundant dietary sources of antioxidants. Supplementary antioxidants, such as vitamins E, C, carotenoids, flavonoids, lipoic acid, selenium and cysteine may provide additional protection (see below).

Boosting your own antioxidant defenses Living beings have evolved sophisticated systems to protect them from free radicals. Of particular importance are the free radical scavenging enzymes: superoxide dismutase (SOD), catalase and glutathione peroxidase. High levels of these enzymes provide extra protection from free radicals. Mutant fruit flies with high levels of SOD have twice the normal life span. Unfortunately, there has been little research to find safe ways to boost the body's levels of antioxidant enzymes. Melatonin has been shown to raise the levels of glutathione peroxidase and to direct antioxidant activity as well. Some researchers believe that the weakening of antioxidant defenses with age is partly due to a dramatic decline in melatonin production.

Oxidative training Another known way to improve the efficiency of the free radical scavenging systems is through "oxidative training." The rationale here is simple. A moderate, short-term increase in free radical formation stimulates the production of free radical scavenging enzymes without doing much harm to the body. The resulting high level of the antioxidant enzymes lasts longer that the initial offense. The phenomenon when a controlled, repeated exposure to higher levels of free radicals markedly stimulates the production of free radical scavenging enzymes may be responsible for some of the benefits of hyperbaric oxygen and other biooxidative treatments. However, excessive exposure to oxygen, hydrogen peroxide or other oxidizing chemicals is dangerous and may cause irreversible damage to tissues.

A safer and a more enjoyable method of "oxidative training" is exercise. Exercise speeds up the burning of fuel, temporarily increasing the formation of free radicals and stimulating the production of antioxidant enzymes. To achieve health benefits, exercise should be regular, 3 to 6 times a week for 30-60 minutes - but not excessive. Too much exercise generates a heavy stream of free radicals that can't be adequately neutralized by the body's defenses, ultimately leading to faster aging.

Reducing stress Stress unleashes a flood of free radicals that can severely damage body tissues. In the initial phases, the body attempts to boost antioxidant defenses to counter the increase in free radical formation. Severe or prolonged stress, however, eventually depletes antioxidant resources leading to extensive and sometimes irreversible cell damage. Neutralizing excess free radicals protects the body from much of this stress-related damage. For instance, stress-induced peptic ulceration in animals can be prevented by potent antioxidants. The first step in reducing stress-related free radical damage is to avoid stressful situations. Second, one may try to modify psychological reactivity through meditation and other relaxation techniques. Increasing your body's intake of antioxidant nutrients during stressful times (unless you are already on high doses of antioxidants) will also help protect you from stress-induced free radical damage.

Adaptogens The agents mitigate stress response and were shown to dramatically decrease the amount of free radicals formed during stress.

ANTIOXIDANT NUTRIENTS AND FOOD SUPPLEMENTS

There are a tremendous variety of antioxidants found in nature -- strong and weak, large and small, essential and nonessential, white and colored. Some essential antioxidants also have other important roles in the body as well. For instance, vitamin C is also required for the synthesis of collagen, the key structural protein in skin and bones. Vitamin A is essential for vision and normal growth of cell in intestinal lining and skin.

An extremely important chemical property of an antioxidant is its solubility in water and fat. Living organisms have two types of internal environment, watery or fatty. Both extracellular and intracellular space are watery. Cell membranes and lipoproteins (small globules circulating in the blood) are fat based. Water-soluble antioxidants are effective mainly in extra and intracellular fluid. Whereas fat-soluble antioxidants protect membranes and lipoproteins. Both types of antioxidants are needed to create an effective shield for the entire body against free radicals.

Water soluble	Fat soluble	Water and fat soluble
Vitamin C Cysteine Methionine Selenium Glutathione	Vitamin E Vitamin A Carotenes Lycopene Coenzyme Q10	Lipoic acid Melatonin Some polyphenols Some flavonoids

Table 13. Solubility of antioxidants

Vitamin C

Vitamin C is a key water soluble antioxidant vitamin. In addition, it is a co-factor in the synthesis of collagen and has a major role in supporting normal immune function. In the US, recommended daily allowance of vitamin C is 60 milligrams, which is enough to prevent scurvy, a vitamin C deficiency disease. Food sources of vitamin C include: citrus fruits, melons, berries, peppers, potatoes, cabbage, broccoli, tomatoes, and fortified cereals. The possible health benefits of generous vitamin C intake include: lower risk of atherosclerosis and cataracts, improved immune function and better wound healing. The amount required to maintain optimal health remains a controversial subject. Linus Pauling, the Nobel laureate and a pioneer of vitamin C research, recommended very high doses - one thousand grams per day. However, recent research indicates that doses as low as 500 mg may under some circumstances promote rather then inhibit free radical formation. As of now, the best strategy is to obtain vitamin C from food, e.g., by drinking orange juice. Considering the conflicting data on vitamin C, we believe that supplements should not exceed 250 mg a day.

<u>Risks concerning high doseage</u> High doses of vitamin C may interfere with tests for hidden blood in stool. A test is sometimes used to diagnose certain gastrointestinal diseases and colon cancer. Since vitamin C increases the absorption and retention of iron, high doses should not be taken by people with genetic conditions such as hemochromatosis or talassemia, who are predisposed to iron overload. Vitamin C in high doses can also interfere with some cancer treatments. Very high doses (tens of grams) may cause diarrhea and gastrointestinal distress. Gastrointestinal side effects may be minimized by taking vitamin C in the form of calcium ascorbate.

Vitamin E

Vitamin E is a principal fat soluble antioxidant that exists within the body. It protects cell membranes and lipoproteins, structures that are especially vulnerable to free radicals because they contain highly reactive unsaturated fatty acids.

In several studies, high doses of vitamin E were shown to inhibit the progression of atherosclerosis and reduce the risk of heart disease and stroke. Arterial plaque growth depends on capturing LDL particles from the bloodstream. When LDL are oxidized, they become sticky and accumulate in the plaque at a much higher rate. Vitamin E effectively inhibits LDL oxidation, thereby blocking atherosclerosis progression.

Recent evidence indicates that vitamin E can slow down aging of the brain. Brain tissue is rich in unsaturated fatty acids which must be protected from the large amounts of free radicals generated by the fast metabolism of neurons. In a recent study, patients with moderate

Alzheimer's disease were given 2,000 IU's of vitamin E per day for two years. In those who received vitamin E, the progression of the disease was 52% slower than in the control group.

The RDA for vitamin E is 30 mgs per day. Food sources of vitamin E include vegetable oil, nuts, wheat germ, whole grains, and green leafy vegetables. The doses of vitamin E which have showed health benefits in various clinical studies ranged from 400 to 2,000 IU's a day. It is extremely difficult, if not impossible, to obtain such amounts even if you "pig out "constantly on vitamin E rich foods.

Potential side effects of high doses High doses may increase the action of anticoagulant drugs and interfere with absorption of vitamin K which has a role in blood clotting. Vitamin E supplements should not be taken before surgery.

Selenium

Selenium is an essential component of a key antioxidant enzyme, glutathione peroxidase. This enzyme inactivates the toxic lipid peroxides. Selenium deficiency has been linked to heart disease. To prevent deficiencies, recommended intakes are 70 micrograms for men and 55 micrograms per day for women. Also shown to reduce the risk of several types of cancer, most experts recommend 200 mg of selenium a day for cancer prevention. Food sources of selenium include seafood, organ meats and some grains and cereals.

Potential side effects of high doses As with many other trace minerals, selenium intake has a relatively narrow margin of safety. High doses or environmental exposure may cause gastrointestinal, neurological and other problems. Doses above 200 mg a day are not recommended.

Cysteine and methionine

Cysteine and methionine are sulphur-based amino acids. In addition to being the basic structural units of proteins, these amino acids act as antioxidants and also facilitate the removal of heavy metals from the body. Cysteine is also a part of glutathione, which is the primary water-soluble antioxidant inside cells. Methionine is an essential amino acid. It cannot be produced by the body and must come from food. Cysteine can be synthesized in the body from methionine and is considered conditionally essential. This means that cysteine may become essential if the body's supply of methionine is limited. Most protein rich foods contain some amount of methionine and cysteine. Good sources of sulphur-containing amino acids include beans, fish, liver, eggs, brewers yeast and nuts.

The content of methionine and cysteine in the body appears to decline with age. A diet supplement with these amino acids increases life span in mice. This suggests that by maintaining optimal levels of sulphur-containing amino acids in humans, it may provide some health and longevity benefits. Cysteine and methionine are available over-the-counter in most health food stores.

LYCOPENE

Lycopene, found in tomatoes is a red pigment that has recently come to the attention of medical researchers. It has been shown to reduce the risk of several common cancers, including prostate, colon and lung cancer. This effect is attributed to the potent antioxidant activity of lycopene. The best way to get a generous supply of lycopene is to consume plenty of foods containing cooked tomatoes. Raw tomatoes are not as good a source of lycopene because high temperatures are needed to release lycopene from plant cells. Choose tomato sauce for all your pastas! Lycopene is also available as a supplement, although you may find it prohibitively expensive.

LIPOIC ACID

Lipoic acid is a conditionally essential nutrient required by the cell for producing energy from carbohydrates and other fuels. It is also an effective antioxidant and a chelator of heavy metals. The body can synthesize lipoic acid in modest amounts but the production may fall short of requirements in situations such as stress or illness. As with many other key substances in the body, levels of lipoic acid decline with age.

Lipoic acid is unique among antioxidants in its versatility. It is both water and fat-soluble, capable of protecting all body tissues and compartments. It is effective against most types of free radicals, including the superoxide, anion, hyproxyl radical, singlet oxygen, and hydrogen peroxide. It also chelates (binds to and neutralizes) the ions of metals that catalize free radical formation (iron, copper, cadmium, lead and mercury). Lipoic acid was shown in various animal studies to markedly reduce the rate of LDL oxidation and increase the supply of oxygen to the brain and heart.

Lipoic acid also lowers blood glucose and thereby reduces the impact of another aging mechanism, glycation and cross-linking. In one study with rats suffering from type II diabetes, lipoic acid improved insulin sensitivity and glucose utilization by 30% - 50% and reduced plasma insulin and free fatty acids by 15% - 17%. Several studies in humans showed lipoic acid to improve diabetic neuropathy.

Unfortunately, the best dietary source of lipoic acid is red meat which is relatively high in saturated fat and cholesterol. Supplements may be a healthier way to increase one's intake of lipic acid. For healthy people, the recommended dose of lipoic acid is 100 - 400 mg a day. In diabetic neuropathy studies, the dose of 600 mg a day was the most effective. At these doses, lipoic acid appears to be safe.

Flavonoids

Flavonoids are a diverse group of plant pigments with antioxidant properties. These substances are responsible for the color of many fruits, vegetables and flowers. Aside from being potent antioxidants, some flavonoids have anti-allergenic, anti-carcinogenic, anti-viral and anti-inflammatory properties.

Over 4,000 flavonoids have been characterized and classified. Grape seed extract was found to be one of the best sources of flavonoids with a potent "broad-spectrum" antioxidant capacity. Many flavonoids have a unique affinity to a particular organ, tissue or cell type and therefore may be ideal for targeted prevention or treatment.

For instance, flavonoids from the plant **Silybum marianum** (milk thistle) are potent antioxidants with a strong affinity for the liver. Extracts from *Silybum marianum* can protect the liver from various kinds of toxic damage as well as speed up recovery from liver infections.

Flavonoids from another remarkable plant, **Ginko biloba** have an affinity with the central nervous system. Ginko biloba flavonoids protect neurons from oxidative damage and improve blood flow to the brain. Several studies have shown that Ginko biloba extracts improve memory and learning in the elderly. It may slow the progression of Alzheimer's disease and may even reverse this disease in some cases. Ginkgo biloba flavonoids are among the most promising substances to combat aging of the human brain.

Flavonoids from grape seeds, Ginkgo biloba and Silybum marianum are unavailable in common foods and have to be purchased as supplements. However, there are a vast variety of flavonoids found in common fruits and vegetables - some of them are well known, others barely known and still others, yet to be discovered. One well-known example is Quercetin; a flavonoid found in citrus fruits. It is both an antioxidant and anti-allergen. Consuming generous amounts of various fruits and vegetables is a good way to get a wide variety of beneficial flavonoids.

Vitamin A and carotenes

Vitamin A plays a variety of roles in the body and is also an antioxidant. In the immune system it is essential for vision and for growth of epithelial cells in the skin, intestinal lining and other organs. The RDA for vitamin A is 5,000 IUs. Food sources of vitamin A include liver, egg yolks, fortified milk and milk products, and fish oil. As an antioxidant, vitamin A appears somewhat less effective than vitamins C and E.

Carotenes are a group of structurally similar plant pigments. Carotenes are responsible for the yellow and orange colors in plants like carrots, which are rich in a, b and g carotene. Some carotenes, notably b-carotene, can serve as provitamin A, which simply means they can be converted to vitamin A in the body. Many carotenes and carotenoids are potent antioxidants. Thus far, research has focused mainly on b-carotene. These studies, based upon the preventive value of b-carotene supplements, have mixed results. Small doses of b-carotene are a valuable source of vitamin A, especially in those with low vitamin A levels. However, the antioxidant role of b-carotene in the body has been questioned since in some circumstances, b-carotene can actually promote oxidation and free radical formation. Until we know more, supplementing b-carotene as an antioxidant or substitute for vitamin A is not recommended.

Potential side effects of high doses Vitamin A has a high potential for toxicity. Signs of vitamin A excesses include dry skin, vision problems, bone pain, headache and irritability. In children, bone and skin symptoms may persist even after the supplement has been discontinued. In adults, vitamin A toxicity has been reported after routine intakes of over 50,000 IU a day, and toxicity threshold in children may be considerably lower. CAUTION: In pregnant women, doses as low as 25,000 - 50,000 IU have been linked to birth defects.

Green tea polyphenols

Green tea is one of the most readily available and affordable sources of dietary antioxidants. It is rich in polyphenols, a type of flavonoids with strong antioxidant properties. High consumption of green tea may provide a wide variety of health benefits from reduced risk of some cancers to protection of the liver from toxins, as well as the prevention of heart disease, dental caries and gingivitis.

Compared to most other plants, green tea has been extremely well-researched with literally hundreds of studies in animals and dozens in humans. In various animal models pertaining to cancer, green tea extract was shown to inhibit all stages of carcinogenesis and even cause partial regression of some tumors. In particular, green tea appears to block mutations in DNA caused by a wide range of toxins as well as ultraviolet radiation. Most human studies have attempted to correlate green tea and cancer in a given population. The data collected from these studies is indirect and less reliable because there are too many variables to take into account. It appears that heavy consumption of green tea reduces the risk of at least some cancers, particularly of colon, stomach, pancreatic and esophageal malignancies. The effects of green tea may be especially significant in people with an increased risk of cancer.

In an intriguing study, Korean researchers investigated the effects of green tea and coffee consumption in the frequency of sister-chromatid exchange (SCE) in smokers. SCE is the type of mutations that correlates with the risk of cancer. Smokers had a higher SCE frequency than nonsmokers (9.46 vs 7.03). However, smokers who consumed 2 - 3 cups of green tea a day for 6 months had a SCE frequency of only 7.93. In contrast, the equivalent consumption of coffee did not reduce SCE frequency.

Several studies point to the benefits of green tea in cardiovascular disease. Green tea was shown to inhibit the oxidation of LDL and proliferation of vascular smooth muscle, two important factors in the progression of atherosclerosis.

Another remarkable effect of green tea is its ability to inhibit the growth of oral bacteria and improve acid-resistance to tooth enamel. These effects help prevent gingivitis and dental caries.

Now would be a good time to emphasize the difference between green and black teas. Fresh tea leaves are naturally high in polyphenols, the compounds responsible for most of the health benefits of tea and its extracts. Green tea is prepared in such a way that polyphenols are preserved.

In contrast, the technology of black tea production involves the oxidation of polyphenols. As a result, black tea has about 6 times fewer active polyphenols than green tea.

Most evidence indicates that to obtain significant health benefits, one should consume at least 8-10 cups of green tea a day. (It seems that people with a greater risk of developing cancer, smokers, for example, may benefit from amounts as little as 2-3 cups per day.) For some people, a complete switch from coffee and soda to green tea may suffice to achieve the required amount. Others may choose to take supplements of green tea extract available in health food stores. Keep in mind that any brewed tea, green or black, contains caffeine. However, the amount of caffeine in commercial green tea extracts is usually low.

Coenezyme Q10

Coenezyme Q10 (CoQ10) plays two important roles: First, it's an essential part of the cellular respiration system located in the mitochondria, and secondly, it is a good antioxidant. CoQ10 improves both the rate and efficiency of energy production and protects mitochondria from free radicals. The body can produce CoQ10, but many factors, including age, illness, cholesterol-lowering drugs, and malnutrition, can impair this ability. CoQ10 is sometimes called a biomarker of aging because its level correlates so well with aging and degenerative-diseases. In one study, CoQ10 supplementation increased life expectancy in mice by 50%. A large number of studies clearly demonstrate the efficiency of CoQ10 in congestive heart failure and other diseases of heart muscle. Other conditions that appear to be helped by CoQ10 include hypertension, decreased immunity, and muscular atrophy. The doses of CoQ10 found effective in treatment of established disease range from 100 to 300 mg per day. In healthy people 30-100 mg a day is generally recommended.

Melatonin

Melatonin is a hormone produced by the pineal gland in the brain. Among other things, it is also an antioxidant. We discuss the physiology and use of melatonin in detail in Chapter 6.

GUIDELINES FOR ANTIOXIDANT INTAKE

As you can see from the previous list, there are quite a few antioxidant nutrients. Should all be taken as supplements? Should you attempt to obtain them all from food or is there an optimal combination of selected nutrients that provides a good coverage for overall antioxidant protection, health and longevity benefits?

Unfortunately, there is no straight answer. Most of the research on the health effects of antioxidants has been done on animals. While animal data may suggest human benefits, it would be foolish make any firm recommendations without long-term human studies. Presently, the number of human studies on antioxidants don't amount to much. Most of them have focused on a single nutrient. A single nutrient approach reduces the number of variables in the study and helps arrive at conclusive results. More studies are required to determine the optimal combination of antioxidant nutrients for maximal benefits. To some degree, the burden of choice lies with the reader. However, here are the general guidelines.

The safest and perhaps the most enjoyable way to obtain a wide array of antioxidants is to consume foods high in fruits and vegetables. This has added benefits. Fruits and vegetables are rich in other beneficial nutrients and phytochemicals. The diversity of antioxidants found in fruits and vegetables help protect all tissues and cellular structures from different types of free radicals. Eating plenty of fruits and vegetables may sound rather dull and boring, but this advice is not only supported by scientific evidence, but also mothers around the world. Studies have consistently demonstrated that a diet high in fruits and vegetables reduces the risk of degenerative-diseases including: cancer, heart disease, hypertension and diabetes. Current guidelines of the National Cancer Institute and National Academy of Sciences suggest eating at least 2-4 servings of fruit and 3-5 servings of vegetables a day.

Replace your coffee, black tea and sodas with green tea. Remember that green tea also contains caffeine.

If you choose to take antioxidants in supplement form, select at least one water-soluble and at least one fat-soluble antioxidant. If you choose to take a single antioxidant, lipoic acid may be a good choice as it is both fat and water-soluble.

Many antioxidants have affinities for specific organs or other physiological beneficial activities. If you have a specific health condition, find out if there are antioxidants that show positive effects on your condition. For example, CoQ10 has been shown to improve heart failure and hypertension. **Ginko biloba** extract has been demonstrated to improve memory and slow the progression of Alzheimer's disease.

Of course, read as much information as you can on new antioxidant research.

CHAPTER 23

REWINDING THE AGING CLOCK

There is now enough evidence to safely say that there is a central aging clock in the brain. More precisely, this program resides in the area of the brain called the hypothalmus. Another key role of the hypothalamus is to pace the body's development from birth to maturity by gradually shifting its homeostasis in the direction that favors growth and reproduction. Unfortunately, this shifting does not stop after reaching maturity. It keeps right on going, becoming an important factor in aging and age-related diseases. In other words, the developmental program run by the hypothalamus becomes an aging program. In simple terms, it is an aging clock.

The so-called central aging clock is both cause for concern and comfort. The aging process and life span are both controlled in part by this clock. However, we already know enough about this fascinating mechanism to slow it down or in some cases wind it back a bit.

Having started in the Fifties as nothing more than a hypothesis, Dilman's concept has evolved into a theory substantiated by numerous studies. Since the key concept in Dilman's theory is that the hypothalamus gradually loses its sensitivity to hormonal and metabolic feedback from the rest of the body, it causes shifts in the body's homeostasis. This change in the sensitivity of the hypothalamus acts as a mechanism that sets the pace for both the body's development and decline.

The best way to prove a theory scientifically is by making a prediction based on it and to test it experimentally. Dilman's theory maintains that if the sensitivity of the hypothalamus to feedback signals is restored, the aging clock can be rewound, leading to longer life and fewer age-related diseases. That's precisely what happened in a variety of animal studies. When rodents are given drugs that improve the sensitivity of the hypothalamus to feedback signals (e.g., deprenyl, L-DOPA) their life span increases by up to 50% or more. Whether improving the sensitivity of the hypothalamus will produce such dramatic effects in humans has yet to be determined. However, we do know that humans also lose the sensitivity of the hypothalamus with age. This is especially important when you take into consideration that the mechanism for the central aging clock in humans is the same as in other mammals, including rats and mice.

The central aging clock causes a variety of shifts in many body systems. The ones most important to longevity and disease prevention are the changes in how the body utilizes energy and how it reacts to stress. In addition, the central aging clock seems to be partly responsible for the age-related decline in some "youth" hormones, particularly growth hormone and DHEA.

Based on our current understanding, the "rewinding strategy" should restore the sensitivity of the hypothalamus to feedback signals from the body. Such signals include the blood levels of stress steroids, glucose, sex hormones, and others. In addition, measures that reverse the age-related disturbances in the body's energy utilization and stress response will also reduce the negative impact of the central aging clock.

"Health passport"

The central aging clock causes us to grow and mature and later contributes to our aging. If this program didn't exist, it would be impossible for us to develop into adults. The problem is that this program doesn't shut down after we've reached maturity. The ideal scenario would be to let the central aging clock take care of its responsibilities for development in the first twenty to twenty-five years of life and then shut it down. While it is not yet possible to stop the central

Key homeostasis shifts driven by central aging clock	Resulting changes in physiological parameters	Resulting changes in physiological parameters
Abnormal energy utilization	• Impaired glucose tolerance • High blood cholesterol, LDL and triglycerides • Excess insulin • Impaired appetite regulation	• Impaired glucose tolerance • High blood cholesterol, LDL and triglycerides • Excess insulin • Impaired appetite regulation
Abnormal response to stress	• Excessive secretion of stress steroids (cortisol) during stress • Excessive secretion of stress steroids in the absence of stressors • Excess of stress steroid exacerbates most of the above negative changes in energy utilization	• Excessive secretion of stress steroids (cortisol) during stress • Excessive secretion of stress steroids in the absence of stressors • Excess of stress steroid exacerbates most of the above negative changes in energy utilization
Abnormal regulation of reproductive function	• High levels of the hormones that regulate or affect reproductive organs, such as FSH, LH and prolactin	• High levels of the hormones that regulate or affect reproductive organs, such as FSH, LH and prolactin

Table 14. Some homeostatic changes linked to the central aging clock.

clock at maturity, there are ways to slow it down or even temporarily reverse it.

Before we go any further you should have a rough idea of its timing, i.e., how far one's clock is from the ideal point. The ideal point in time is when you were twenty to twenty-five-years-old. Perhaps there is no need to do anything yet or maybe you have no time to waste.

The mechanism of the central aging clock is the gradual loss of sensitivity of the hypothalamus to feedback signals, so to check the time on the central aging clock, one must send a signal to the hypothalamus and measure the magnitude of the response. This is indeed done in research studies and sometimes in clinical practice.

Measuring the response of the hypothalamus to a dozen or more feedback signals provides an adequate assessment of the time on one's central aging clock. Unfortunately, this approach is impractical and inaccessible outside clinical studies. As an alternative to assessing the state of the central clock, Dilman put forth the concept of "Health passports." He noticed that a profile consisting of several key physiological parameters correlated well with the time on the central aging clock. He called this profile a health passport because a good health passport indicated high chances of long life and freedom from degenerative-diseases.

Ideally, the health passport should be determined at twenty to twenty-five years of age and considered the norm for that person. Monitoring changes in the health passport would indicate how far the central aging clock has advanced. The goal of an intervention strategy would be to maintain or restore a normal health passport; i.e., one you had at twenty-five. If you are past that ideal age, it should aim at achieving the values in a typical normal health passport.

For a basic health passport, Dilman suggested that the following be monitored:

- Body weight and body composition (percentage of lean and fat body mass); distribution of fat and waist to hip ratio (central versus peripheral distribution of fat);
- Blood levels of cholesterol, LDL, HDL, and triglycerides (lipid profile);
- Oral glucose tolerance with simultaneous measurement of fasting and 2-hour insulin levels and glycated hemoglobin (metabolism of carbohydrates);
- Blood levels of TSH and T3 (metabolic rate);
- Blood FSH in women and testosterone in men (indicators of the reproductive aspect of the aging clock);
- Arterial blood pressure.

The basic parameters are easily monitored in most people. No change in a health passport indicates that the central aging clock is advancing at a slow pace. Tests for the basic health passport can be routinely done by family physicians. Body composition and fat distribution can be determined by either a doctor or a nutritionist. There are other tests that can determine the pace of the central aging clock with greater accuracy (testing blood levels of IGF-1 and DHEA sulfate). If your physician has an interest in anti-aging medicine, he or she may agree to perform these additional tests. The results of all tests should be compared with either your own results at age twenty-five or, if unavailable, with typical values for twenty-five-year-old people. The greater the difference, the later the time on your central aging clock.

SLOWING DOWN THE CENTRAL AGING CLOCK THROUGH NUTRITION AND LIFESTYLE

DON'T STUFF YOUR FACE

Consumption of excess calories and obesity accelerate the aging process in several ways. Dramatic life extension seen in animal experiments with caloric restriction appears to be partly due to the effects of reduced food intake on the hypothalamus, the core of the aging clock. Based on today's knowledge, the amount of calories consumed should be consistent with obtaining an optimal body weight and youthful body composition.

It is important to note that being overweight seems to accelerate the central aging clock. Conversely, restricting caloric intake slows it down. However, as we discussed earlier, a semi-starvation diet is not a viable option in humans.

MELATONIN

Evidence indicates that melatonin can improve the sensitivity of the hypothalamus to feedback signals, in particular, the levels of corticosteroids and sex hormones. In essence, this means that melatonin helps rewind the central aging clock, which may account for some of the many beneficial effects of this hormone.

Hit the Gym Instead of the Fridge

Exercise does not affect the central clock directly, but, it does improve carbohydrate tolerance, reduces insulin excess and raises HDL. Exercise is also valuable as a stress reduction tool.

Chromium

Chromium is similar to exercise in that it too improves insulin sensitivity, reduces blood glucose levels and improves one's lipid profile. In plain English, it neutralizes some of the negative metabolic effects of the central aging clock. Chromium increases life span in rats. The physiological effects of chromium are largely due to its ability to increase the responsiveness of cells to insulin. Prolonged cultivation of soil may deplete its chromium content so the food you eat may also be depleted as well.

In addition, most food processing methods lose as much as 80% of their chromium content. Marginal chromium deficiency may go unnoticed, and has become a wide spread phenomenon in our society that may contribute to the development of noninsulin-dependent diabetes as well as other age-related diseases.

Most chromium salts are poorly absorbed in the GI tract and lack any biological activity. Chromium picolinate and chromium nicotinate are relatively inexpensive and highly bioavailable chromium salts commonly used as chromium supplements. Experts recommend 200 mg a day. Larger doses, especially above 600 mg a day, are not recommended and may be toxic.

Keeping neurotransmitter levels high

Neurotransmitters are chemicals that transmit messages between neurons in the brain. Efficient communication between neurons requires certain levels of neurotransmitters. Low levels of neurotransmitters are often associated with such conditions as depression and Parkinson's disease. The central aging clock is dependent on neurotransmitters, as is the rest of the central nervous system. If the hypothalamus' levels of neurotransmitters decrease, its sensitivity to feedback signals from the body also decrease. The result is the speeding up of the central aging clock.

Animal studies show that treatments which raise the levels of neurotransmitters in the hypothalamus extend life span and reduce the risk of age-related diseases. Conversely, experimental lowering of the level of neurotransmitters has the opposite effect.

In humans, the condition most commonly associated with low levels of neurotransmitters is depression. In depression, several areas of the brain are depleted of neurotransmitters including the hypothalamus. This situation is likely to speed up the central aging clock. Alleviating depression often raises brain levels of neurotransmitters and may possibly slow down the aging clock. Interestingly enough, one of the most consistent findings in the study of centenarians is a high level of emotional well-being and excellent coping ability - the opposites of depression.

Avoiding and counteracting stress

Stress is a major factor in accelerating the pace of the central aging clock. The stress response is instigated by the hypothalamus, the same part of the brain that acts as the central aging clock. Whenever the hypothalamus is required to maintain a prolonged stress response, it readjusts itself in such a way as to become less sensitive to future feedback signals. This accelerates the central aging clock. In addition, large amounts of free radicals produced by stress can damage the neurons in the hypothalamus, pushing the aging clock even further ahead.

Drugs that may slow down the central aging clock

A number of prescription drugs are capable of raising the sensitivity of the hypothalamus to feedback signals and thus slow down the central aging clock. In animals, these drugs produce a significant extension of life span and decrease the incidence of age-related diseases. Although none of these drugs has been approved by the FDA for anti-aging purposes, they have been successfully used to treat a number of other conditions. Some physicians who specialize in anti-aging medicine prescribe these drugs on a regular basis.

Our general recommendation is to use natural supplements rather than synthesized drugs for anti-aging purposes because substances from natural sources tend to produce fewer side effects.

On the other hand, synthetic drugs may in some cases produce more profound anti-aging effects than their natural alternatives. We believe that current information on anti-aging treatments is insufficient to warrant extensive use of synthetic drugs. It is quite possible in the future these and other drugs will become a part of the standard anti-aging regimen approved by the FDA and practiced by family physicians.

Below we discuss several drugs that have the potential to neutralize the effects of the central aging clock. We believe that anyone seriously interested in life extension should have a working knowledge of all the option modern science has to offer. Keep in mind that these drugs can cause serious side effects in sensitive individuals or when used improperly. None of these drugs should be taken without approval and close supervision of a physician familiar with anti-aging medicine. In addition, be sure to read all instructions, dosage recommendations, side effects, cautions, warnings, and risks associated with their use. Some people may be at a higher risk of side effects than others. Your doctor should be the one to determine if your medical history and current physical state are compatible with the use of any particular drug. Your doctor should also determine the correct dosage and supervise your treatment.

L-DEPRENYL

Deprenyl is the drug with a remarkable anti-aging potential. It dramatically extends life span in laboratory animals, even when treatment starts late in life. In one study, deprenyl administration to old rats increased the life expectancy by 34%.

Deprenyl seems to attack several mechanisms of aging at once. First, it acts by inhibiting the enzyme monoamine oxidase type B in the brain which results in higher levels of neurotransmitters in the hypothalamus and sets the central aging clock back. Second, it stimulates antioxidant defenses in the brain by increasing the synthesis of superoxide dismutase, a key free radical-scavenging enzyme. Finally, deprenyl stimulates the synthesis of melatonin by the pineal gland.

Deprenyl increases both life expectancy and functional capacity in Parkinson's disease patients.

L-DOPA

L-dopa is a precursor of the neurotransmitters dopamine and norepinephrine. L-dopa is similar to deprenyl in respect to resetting the central aging clock by raising the levels of these neurotransmitters in the hypothalamus. L-dopa markedly increases the life span of laboratory animals and restores reproductive function in old female rats. L-dopa is also a very effective growth hormone releaser. In one study, 0.5 gm of L-dopa increased GH levels of healthy men over sixty to those of young adults.

In many cases, L-dopa improves body composition, promoting muscle gain and fat loss. L-dopa also improves stamina and motor coordination, and is effective for Parkinson's disease.

HYDERGINE

Hydergine is a drug commonly used for age-related decline in cognitive function and is often prescribed for Alzheimer's disease and other types of dementia. Hydergine has numerous effects on the brain, including: improved protein synthesis increased oxygen supply, and increased formation of interneuronal connections. The drug seems to work by stimulating the production of neurotransmitters dopamine and norepinephrine and similarly to L-dopa. Hydergine stimulates growth hormone release in people of all ages. Several studies showed hydergine to improve learning, memory, cognitive ability and mood. It appears that benefits of hydergine also include improving the sensitivity of the hypothalamus to feedback signals. In other words, rewinding the aging clock.

PHENYTOIN

Phenytoin (Dilantin) was shown to be beneficial in a remarkably wide range of conditions including; epilepsy, neurological pain, depression, anxiety, ulcers, asthma, mental deterioration and even baldness. Its action is not fully understood.

In many studies, phenytoin had a positive affect on the central aging clock, improving the sensitivity of the hypothalamus to feedback signals, leading to a more youthful metabolism and better hormonal balance. In particular, phenytoin was shown to increase the levels of growth hormone, decrease levels of stress steroids and reduce insulin excess. Rodents treated with phenytoin had longer life spans and longer reproductive periods. In some postmenopausal female animals, phenytoin restored reproductive function. One study reported that epileptic patients on long-term phenytoin therapy had a decreased incidence of cancer.

CHAPTER 24

R & R FOR MIND AND BODY.

Throughout this book, we've emphasized the damaging effects of chronic stress on health and its relationship to aging. We've also discussed which physiological and biochemical changes in the body favor a greater resistance to stress. In this chapter we'll provide you with some practical ways to minimize stress-related damage to the human body. This includes avoiding stress and minimizing its effects when it can't be avoided.

CHANGING ATTITUDES TOWARDS STRESS

In most cases, psychological stress is not about how bad things really are, but how bad you actually perceive them to be. In a situation you cannot change, the healthiest step to take is a change in attitude, which will enable your body to "dial down" its stress response.

Imagine the following scenario. A boy and his father arrive at a train crossing in a car. The father says, "Oh, darn! Now we'll have to wait for this train to pass." The boy says, "Oh, great! Now we get to watch the train go by." Both father and son share the same experience, only the father is likely to develop a stress response. This doesn't mean that all bad situations should simply be accepted as they are. You can take constructive action to change things. Simply doing something about a situation may be enough to relieve stress.

Otherwise, try to find a positive angle or at least accept the ramifications. In almost all cases, whatever it is, chances are it could have been worse.

BIOFEEDBACK

Biofeedback, a computer-aided technique, teaches a person some control over certain involuntary body functions. A computer or some device that monitors bodily functions helps patients to visualize their physiological parameters such as blood pressure, heartbeat or skin temperature and then learn how to get these values into the desirable range. Initially, biofeedback was a typical "alternative" therapy. However, now that it has become scientifically validated, it's safe to say that it has a "foot" in the medical mainstream. Biofeedback is especially effective in stress reduction and conditions exacerbated by stress, such as migraine headaches and chronic fatigue syndrome. Stress, especially in its initial phase, is associated with rapid heartbeat, elevated blood pressure and coldness of the extremities. Using biofeedback to bring these parameters back to normal will reduce the intensity of the stress response and decrease the release of stress hormones. Many psychiatrists and psychotherapists offer biofeedback in their offices. Home use devices are also available.

REWINDING THE CENTRAL AGING CLOCK

As we age, the stress response usually becomes more intense and prolonged than necessary. It leaves the body secreting excess stress hormones even in the absence of stressors. Metabolically speaking, many older people may be in a state of chronic stress without ever suspecting it.

Exercise

One of the benefits of moderate exercise is stress reduction. Exercise tends to reduce the intensity and duration of the stress response in psychologically stressful situations. A good workout goes a long way to wipe out the tension of a stressful day. In terms of stress and general health, the greatest benefits come from a consistent program of moderately intensive regular exercise. Keep in mind that excessive exercise is a substantial stress and does more damage than good.

Restoring youthful levels of hormones

There is some evidence that decreasing levels of hormones - melatonin, DHEA and growth hormone in particular, contribute to a weakening in stress resistance with age. All of these hormones reduce the damaging effects of stress on the immune system. The growth hormone helps protect the body from the loss of lean body mass caused by stress. Melatonin appears to improve the responsiveness of the hypothalamus to signals that shut down the stress response. Steps to help restore youthful levels of these hormones are discussed in Chapter 23.

Relieving depression

One of the diagnostic hallmarks of depression is an abnormal response to stress. In depression, the body is often unable to shut down stress responses, even when they are no longer necessary. This creates a state of chronic stress. Relieving depression usually reverses the situation (see Chapter 9).

ADAPTOGENS

Adaptogens are a group of substances that increase the body's ability to adapt to adverse conditions. Adaptogens improve resistance to both acute and chronic stress and minimize stress-related damage. Chapter 14 is devoted entirely to the benefits of adaptogens.

ANTIOXIDANTS

Stress causes a dramatic increase in the levels of free radicals. Some of the damage can be offset by supplementary oxidants (Chapter 12). In fact, supplementary antioxidants appear to provide more benefits during stress then any other time.

VITAMINS AND MINERALS

Some nutrients are used up or excreted at an accelerated rate during serious periods of stress. High levels of stress hormone cause increased excretion of potassium and retention of sodium. A healthier balance can usually be maintained through a diet high in potassium and low in sodium. Fruits and vegetables are excellent sources of potassium and are also low in sodium.

Vitamin C, pantothenic acid and vitamin B6 are important in the normal functioning of the adrenal glands which have to pull an extra load during stress. During serious stress these nutrients should be consumed in amounts higher than the RDA. For most people, twice the RDA supplementation is sufficient. However, large doses of B6 (tens of times the RDA, taken for several months) may produce nerve damage and should not be taken.

Relaxation Techniques

Proper relaxation raises the body's threshold of stress response to various psychologically adverse situations. It can also help ease ongoing stress. Relaxation reduces heart rate and blood pressure, decreases perspiration, increases blood flow to internal organs and improves secretion of digestive juices. Blood sugar tends to return to a normal range, the opposite effect of the body's reaction to the initial phase of the stress response.

There are numerous techniques used to achieve a state of relaxation, some more effective than others. Biofeedback is in essence, a relaxation technique. The choice of the best relaxation technique is highly individual, and some trial and error is involved before you arrive at the right choice.

Specific discussion of relaxation techniques go beyond the scope of this book, but numerous books written on the subject offer various alternatives. A popular technique is progressive relaxation based upon alternating tension and relaxation. Most people are completely unaware of whether they are tense or relaxed. In truth, the goal of this technique is to teach awareness muscle relaxation compared to tension. A muscle is first contracted forcefully for a few seconds and then relaxed. This process goes through all the muscles in the body, eventually resulting in a state of deep relaxation. This procedure is usually started with the muscles of the face and neck and then continued downward along the body. Some people found it easier to relax by imagining that their limbs are becoming heavy and warm. Others imagine themselves in some ideally peaceful and agreeable place like a remote tropical island. Most experts recommend at least 10 minutes each day be devoted to relaxation.

ENHANCING YOUR STRESS-LIMITING SYSTEMS

The body has a number of built-in mechanisms that curtail or limit stress induced damage. We have discussed these systems in detail in Chapter 20. Some of these systems can be safely enhanced with nutrients; in particular, growth hormone whose release is increased during stress. Growth hormone has a role in reducing the damaging effects of stress on lean tissue and the immune system. The release of growth hormone can be further enhanced by nutrients.

The stress response is also followed by the release of enkephalins and endorfins, morphine-like substances naturally produced by the body. Enkephalins and endorfins are also capable of reducing damage caused by stress. The amino acid DL-phenylalanine increases the levels of enkephalins by inhibiting the enzyme that degrades them. DL-phenylalanine appears to be especially effective in relieving stress associated with pain and depression (see Chapter 17).

CHAPTER 25

"YOUTH HORMONES"
YOU'RE ONLY YOUNG TWICE.

As we discussed in Chapter 5, aging is associated with changes in the levels of many major hormones. It was long believed that these hormonal shifts were purely a consequence of aging and there was nothing that could be done about it. As it turned out, some hormonal changes may actually stimulate the aging process. Conversely, reversal may help counteract it.

Three major hormones undergo a dramatic decline with age: growth hormone (GH), melatonin and DHEA. Low levels of each may contribute to the aging process and the development of degenerative-diseases. Numerous animal experiments and some short-term human studies indicate that restoring GH, melatonin and DHEA levels to their youthful states may help slow down the aging process. Unfortunately, no long-term studies have been conducted.

The state of affairs with GH, melatonin and DHEA are currently similar to the situation associated with estrogen replacement therapy thirty years ago. We now know that some studies show that estrogen replacement in women provides a small but significant increase in life span and reduces the risk of heart disease and osteoporosis. Conversely, it increases the risk of breast cancer, so most doctors recommend that postmenopausal women at risk for heart disease should take estrogens while those at risk should not. The final verdict on GH, melatonin and DHEA may prove even more complicated. At this point, possible anti-aging benefits of these hormones are nothing more than educated guesses.

Does this mean that everyone should wait 30 years before they have the knowledge to evaluate the data? Not necessarily, but the decision to restore youthful levels of key hormones is a matter of personal philosophy. Some physicians actively treat many of their patients with GH, DHEA, and melatonin. Others do it occasionally, and very cautiously, while still others prefer to wait until all data is in. Many people self-medicate as a result of media hype, friends' advice or their own analysis of current research. If you decide to take action, you should first talk to your doctor, making sure you don't have any conditions that place you at risk to adverse side effects.

Restoring GH levels

Possible benefits, side effects and general precautions.

In animals, GH was shown to increase life span and delay the onset of age-related diseases. Available human studies indicate that restoring youthful levels of GH may provide a number of health and life extension benefits including but not limited to the following (see Chapter 5 for a detailed discussion):

- Improved body composition: loss of fat tissue, and increase in muscle mass,
- Enhanced immunity,
- Elevated mood, greater sense of well-being,
- Better cardiovascular performance, including patients with congestive heart failure,
- Increased physical performance,
- Better wound healing, shorter hospital stays after surgery, and
- Reversal of age-related atrophy of organs, including heart, kidneys, liver, spleen, and skin.

For all its benefits, both proven and unproved, GH replacement must be approached with common sense and reason. Excessive amounts of GH can cause serious damage. Acromegaly is a rare condition that develops when the body produces too much GH: the signs and symptoms of acromegaly include enlargement of joints and joint pain, thickening of skin, coarsening of facial features, soft tissue swelling in the hands and feet, carpal tunnel syndrome, edema and development of deep husky voice. Some of these side effects were reported in individuals treated with high dose injections of recombinant human growth hormone (produced via the methods of genetic engineering). Experts believe that side effects are likely if GH levels are significantly above those of healthy young people. Such levels were seen in some high dose GH replacement studies and were associated with frequent side effects. When GH levels are restored to the physiological norm for young adults, the side effects are uncommon, but still possible. In this context, it is paramount that a person embarking on GH replacement therapy should have their IGF-1 levels checked. (IGF-1 is one of the major mediators GH action in the body). GH levels undergo dramatic fluctuations during the day because it is released in pulses, and as a result a single measurement of GH may not reflect the real picture. On the other hand, IGF-I levels are relatively steady and reflect the total amount of GH produced in the body.

There are two approaches to raising GH levels. One is simply to inject the GH solution. The advantage of this approach is that you reliably introduce a known quantity of GH into the body. The disadvantages, however, include high cost, significant risk of side effects, and the need for regular injections.

Another approach is to jolt the pituitary into releasing more GH. Along with GH therapy, changes in diet and exercise habits provide additional stimulation. The advantages of this method are lower costs, lower risk of side effects and convenient oral administration. However, the true disadvantage to this method is high individual variability in response to GH-releasers. While some people release enough GH to restore youthful levels, others may have only a slight increase in GH production. Also, the pituitary gland's response to some GH-releasers as well as exercise may decrease with age.

We need to emphasize that GH injection therapy or GH releasers make sense only if GH production is decreased; i.e. (if IGF-I levels are low, which is common after the age of forty and almost universal after sixty). Taking steps to raise GH levels, especially via GH injections, should only be done under strict medical supervision. It is prudent to check IGF-I levels before and during the therapy and be alert to side effects.

Age (years)	Serum IGF-I (ng/ml)
16 - 24	182 - 780
25 - 39	114 - 492
40 - 54	90 - 360
over 55	71 - 290

GH INJECTIONS

Growth hormone is a protein. When GH is taken orally, digestive enzymes destroy a good portion of it, with only negligible amounts making it into the blood stream intact, if any. As a result, oral growth hormone does not produce any significant physiological effects. The only way to get exogenous GH into the bloodstream is by injection. At this point, optimal GH replacement doses and dosing schedules have yet to be clearly defined.

To minimize the risk of side effects, most experts recommend GH doses that raise IGF-1 to levels seen in twenty-five to thirty-five year-old adults. A common recommendation is to start with 0.5 IUs a day (IU of growth hormone is 3 mg), raising it in monthly increments of 0.1-0.25 IUs until desired IGF-1 levels are reached. Doses over 2 IUs are very likely to cause noticeable side effects. Existing studies indicate that a low dose/high frequency administration (small doses twice a day) is a more effective method and produces fewer side effects than a low-frequency high dose injection approach (2-4 times a week).

Indeed, the former regimen mimics more closely the body's own GH production, which occurs daily in short spurts. Older people are more sensitive to GH and generally require less to achieve desirable IGF-1 levels. In most people over sixty, 0.5 IU of GH a day is sufficient.

At this time, the cost of GH is prohibitive for most people. For an average adult, the cost is between $10,000 to $18,000 a year. The cost is likely to go down in the near future as pharmaceutical companies rush into the market, but it does not seem likely that GH will become affordable any time soon.

Another downside of the GH injection approach is that the body's own GH production is inhibited as a result of a negative feedback loop. GH and IGF-1 suppress the signals from the hypothalamus to the pituitary gland to produce GH. A person with diminished but significant GH secretion may lose the ability to produce GH (at least for several weeks) after prolonged GH replacement therapy. This obstacle can be partially circumvented by giving GH injections in cycles, which enables the body's own GH secretion to recover. There is no consensus on the optimal dose cycling, although some physicians recommend ceasing one week every month. Others recommend ceasing one day every week.

Boosting your own GH production

Most people can reap the anti-aging benefits of restored GH and IGF-1 levels without spending a fortune, and with low risk of side effects. This can be achieved through stimulating the pituitary gland to release GH. A number of substances, both natural and synthetic, can jolt the pituitary gland into releasing GH. Exercise and dietary changes can enhance the effects of GH releasers. You'll find an outline for GH enhancement regimen on the next page. For more detailed information see the book, "Grow Young with HGH," by Dr. Ronald Klatz and Carol Kahn.

Nutrients stimulating GH release

GH releasers act upon the pituitary gland to stimulate GH secretion. Many GH releasers are nutrients and can be used either alone or in combination. The ability to respond to GH releasers decreases somewhat with age. Still, in most older people, a significant increase in GH secretion can be achieved.

Arginine

The best known GH releaser is arginine, an essential amino acid which can only be obtained through diet. An intravenous administration of 15-30 grams of arginine is the standard endocrinological test for determining the capacity of the pituitary gland to secrete growth hormone. Individual responses to arginine vary significantly; from no effect to a dramatic rise. Some response to arginine is usually preserved even in advanced old age.

Usage: Arginine may be used alone or in combination with other GH releasers. It should be taken on an empty stomach one hour before exercise and at bedtime. Usual dosage can range from 1.5 to 5 gms. Nausea, diarrhea and stomach upset may occur at higher dosages. People with serious herpes infection should not take arginine because it can stimulate the replication of the virus.

Ornithine

Ornithine is an amino acid structurally close to arginine and can be synthesized from arginine in the body. Ornithine acts similarly to arginine, but at a somewhat higher activity level. Individual responses to ornithine vary as much as for arginine.

Usage: Dosage and side effects are the same as for arginine. Ornithine should be taken at bedtime on an empty stomach.

LYSINE

Lysine is an essential amino acid. Taken alone, it does not significantly affect GH secretion, but it markedly augments the GH-releasing effect of arginine. In one study, Dr. Isidori and colleagues at the University of Rome, found that in young males, a combination of 1,200 mg of arginine and lysine each, was ten times more effective than 1,200 mg of arginine alone. The response to lysine/arginine combination seems to decline with age.

Usage: 1gm on an empty stomach together with arginine before exercise and bedtime.

GLUTAMINE

Glutamine is a conditionally essential amino acid. Normally, the body can synthesize it in sufficient quantities, but under stress the synthesis may fail to meet the required needs. Glutamine is also an effective GH releaser. Studies indicate that the response to glutamine does not significantly diminish with age. Glutamine has a variety of other beneficial effects. It is a key fuel for the cells of the GI tract and helps maintain a healthy intestinal lining and neutralizes some adverse effects to stress, particularly muscle wasting. A correlation has been found between low levels of glutamine and heart disease, diabetes and arthritis.

Usage: 2 gms at bedtime. It appears that both lower and higher doses are less effective.

GLYCINE

This amino acid is not as well researched as other GH-releasers, but at least 2 studies indicate that it does enhance GH secretion, starting with as little as 250 mg.

Usage: 250 mg to 6 gms a day. Glycine is inexpensive and usually very well tolerated.

NIACIN

Niacin is a B vitamin found in 2 main forms, nicotinic acid and niacinamide. Among its many activities is the ability to stimulate GH release. Xanthinol nicotinate is the most potent form of niacin that stimulate GH release, probably because it crosses the blood-brain barrier.

Usage: 200-500 mg a day alone or in combination with other releasers. It may cause transient and harmless flush, but beginning with 100 mg and slowly increasing the dosage can minimize this reaction. Tolerance to flushing usually develops in a few days. High doses of niacin (several grams) are known to dramatically improve lipid profile, lowering LDL and triglycerides and rising HDL. However, high doses of niacin, especially in sustained release form, have been linked to cases of hyperglycemia and liver damage.

GHB

GHB is both a metabolite and a precursor of GABA, an inhibitory neurotransmitter involved, among other things, in limiting stress-related damage (see Chapter 4). As opposed to GABA, GHB easily crosses the blood brain barrier and prompts a number of responses including GH release. In fact, GHB is a very effective GH releaser working by raising dopamine levels in the hypothalamus.

Usage: Low doses of GHB (500-750 gs), safely stimulate GH release without significant side effects. GHB can be combined with other GH releasers. (**The FDA withdrew GHB fromthe U.S. market in 1990**).

At high doses, GHB can cause very deep sleep and muscle spasms, and at very high doses - coma. It should not be taken with alcohol, antidepressants or tranquilizers.

Note: A number of prescription drugs are effective GH releasers. For a review of GH releasing drugs see the book "Grow Young with HGH," by Dr. Ronald Klatz and Carol Kahn.

COMBINING GH RELEASERS

GH releasers are often used in combination because their effec.. are additive and sometimes synergistic. No system to date has been adopted on the optimal combination for any specific age group. One popular combination is agrinine,1-2 gms; ornithine, 1-2 gms; lysine, 1 gm; glutamine, 2 gms; niacin (or xanthinol nicotinate), 0.2-0.5 gms. It is recommended to start with lower dosages and increase them over time to minimize the risk of side effects. Many commercial formulas for GH release are now available, and the new ones are popping up regularly. Because there have been few clinical studies, the effectiveness of most of these formulas is unclear. Check the ingredients to see that at least some of the above GH releasing nutrients are included.

Of particular interest is a recently released formula called Amino-Tropin-6 made by Gero Vita International. It includes GHRP (growth hormone-releasing peptide), arginine, lysine, GABA, and xanthinol nicotinate. GHRP, the formula's key active ingredient, is a short chain of amino acids that simulates the action of GHRH (growth hormone releasing hormone), a hormone that normally stimulates GH release in the body. The company claims that AminoTropin-6 boosts GH secretion by up to 50% without adverse side effects.

GH AND DIET

People who are overweight or obese have lower GH and IGF-1 levels, and are also less responsive to GH releasers. Reducing caloric intake via a balanced high fiber, low-fat diet and reasonable exercise (as discussed in Chapter 21) is the single most important thing one can do to enhance GH secretion.

Some evidence indicates that a high protein diet may modestly increase GH secretion. Ingestion of large amounts of protein raises blood levels of amino acids, including those which stimulate the pituitary to release GH. On the other hand, excess protein puts an undue strain on liver and kidneys, the two organs handling the disposal of excess amino acids. Generally, 10%-20% of total calories should come from protein. People should aim somewhere in the range of 0.8-1.2 gms of protein per kilogram of body weight. However, vigorous physical activity increases protein requirements but most experts believe that higher protein intakes (about 25% of calories from protein or up to two gms per kilogram) are justified with an intense exercise program. When raising your protein intake, select foods rich in high quality protein but low in saturated fat such as fish, lean poultry, low-fat dairy products and soy.

GH AND EXERCISE

Exercise is an effective way to jolt the pituitary gland into releasing growth hormone. The mechanisms of this effect are unclear, but the most plausible hypothesis is that exercise stimulates GH release by raising the levels of endorphins (endogenous morphine-like substances with many functions in the body). The stimulating effect of exercise on GH release declines with age but may remain significant even in very old individuals.

There is an ongoing controversy as to the best type of exercise to enhance GH and IGF-1 levels. Most experts agree that a combination of moderate intensity aerobics, (such as running, race walking or stationary bike), with moderate-to-high intensity weight training provides optimal results for most people. We suggest the following general guidelines:

- Before initiating an exercise program, consult a physician and have a comprehensive sports medicine physical,
- Increase the duration and intensity of exercise, slowly, do not go for high intensity until you are well conditioned,

- Exercise at least every other day for at least half an hour,
- Drink plenty of fluids to avoid dehydration,
- High intensity exercise should be undertaken, initially, under the supervision of a qualified professional.

For detailed information on an exercise program to enhance your GH levels we recommend the book by Dr. Ronald Klatz and Jo Robinson, "Grow Young with hGH."

Restoring melatonin levels

Possible benefits, side effects and general precautions

Melatonin has become one the most popular nutritional supplements in the United States in recent years. In rodents, melatonin extends life span by about 20% and provides protection from some diseases and stress.

As with growth hormone, DHEA and most other "fountain-of-youth" substances, long-term human studies of melatonin are at best sketchy. At this point, it seems that restoring youthful levels of melatonin in middle-aged, and especially older people, may provide some possible and probable health benefits, including, but not limited to the following (see Chapter 6) for a detailed discussion:

- Improved immune function,
- Slowing down of the "central aging clock" in the hypothalamus,
- Protection from free radical damage, especially in the brain,
- Reduction in cancer risk and inhibition of tumor growth,
- Enhancement of anti-cancer therapies,

(with higher than physiological doses of melatonin),
- Improved resistance to stress,
- Better sleep.

As we mentioned, people over forty produce about 1/3 as much melatonin as in their early twenties, whereas individuals aged sixty or older produce only negligible amounts.

Melatonin has little or no acute toxicity, even at doses as high as several gms (a typical supplement contains 3 mg of melatonin per tablet). Short-term, low-dose use of melatonin supplements appears to be safe, but long-term safety has yet to be determined. Adverse side effects are minor and infrequent, the most common being drowsiness. Melatonin should not be taken together with sedatives, tranquilizers, alcohol or psychoactive drugs.

It should be kept in mind that supplements may inhibit the body's natural melatonin production. The release of most hormones is regulated by the negative feedback mechanism, which means that high levels of a hormone inhibit its further release. The administration of supplemental melatonin usually inhibits its natural release. There are few studies to verify how much or for how long supplements inhibit natural release of melatonin. It is possible, however, that prolonged administration of melatonin supplements may impair one's ability to produce their own melatonin. For people under forty who usually produce sufficient amounts of melatonin, this should be a concern. Children and young adults who have very high levels of melatonin should not take supplements unless prescribed by a doctor. There are other people who should not take melatonin for medical or other reasons. If in doubt contact your doctor.

WHO SHOULD NOT TAKE MELATONIN

Children have naturally high levels of melatonin which plays an important role in pacing their development. Use of supplements may inhibit their ability to produce melatonin and may even affect the onset and course of puberty.

Pregnant women and nursing mothers The risks of melatonin in pregnant women has not been studied. Some melatonin can be passed from a nursing mother to an infant through breast milk.

People with autoimmune diseases, such as lupus or rheumatoid arthritis, or severe allergies Melatonin stimulates the immune system, and may exacerbate these conditions.

People taking anti-inflammatory steroids, such as prednisone, or other immunosuppressant medications Melatonin may counteract the effects of these drugs.

People with cancers of the immune system, such as leukemia or lymphoma Melatonin stimulates the immune system, and may exacerbate these conditions.

Women trying to conceive In some women, doses greater than 10 mg may prevent ovulation.

Boosting the body's melatonin production

Starting at puberty, melatonin levels steadily decline, becoming barely detectable after age sixty. Is it possible to maintain or restore youthful levels by stimulating the body's own production like that of growth hormone? The answer is yes, but only to some degree. In a middle-aged person, various life style changes may significantly increase melatonin levels, allowing anyone to take full advantage of its potential benefits without supplements. However, after about age sixty, supplements become the only solution if youthful levels are to be attained.

A number of things can inhibit melatonin production. The most common culprit is the lack of natural light-dark cycle. As we discussed in chapter 14, one of the key functions of melatonin is to regulate sleep-wake cycles. It is secreted in the evening and helps induce sleep. A natural light-dark cycle (bright light during the day and darkness during the night) favors normal secretion of melatonin. Conversely, if the illumination cycle is disturbed, melatonin production declines. Both lack of bright light during the day, and excessive lighting at night inhibit melatonin production. Unfortunately, it is all too common for us to spend most of the day in a dim office and then have bright lights on at home late at night. Studies suggest that for optimal sleep-wake cycle you need to spend at least an hour a day at light levels of outdoor daylight. According to some estimates, only about 5% of adults receive this amount of light exposure. Reading beside a lamp or looking out of a window does not begin to approach the illumination levels of outdoor light. Try spending time outdoors during the day. A stroll or jog in the park or outdoor sport may be a good alternative to workouts in a gym. When in the sun, however, use sunscreen, and sunglasses with UV protection. You can increase your light exposure at home or office by opening your drapes and blinds during the day, and sitting near the window. Minimizing light exposure and getting adequate sleep at night is equally important for optimal melatonin levels.

Several prescription and over-the-counter drugs are another common source that impair natural melatonin production. Among melatonin's enemies are some extremely common medications including aspirin, ibuprofen, beta-blockers, calcium channel blockers, diazepam (Valium), and alprazolam (Xanax).

Do not discontinue any prescribed medication for this reason. Possible health consequences can be far more dangerous than low levels of melatonin. You may discuss with your doctor a possibility of using an alternative drug that won't affect your melatonin levels. You might also consider adding a melatonin supplement to your regimen. Caffeine, tobacco and alcohol depresses melatonin levels, as well. Let preserving your melatonin be yet another reason for curtailing or quitting any or all of these habits.

Stress has a two-way relationship with melatonin levels. While melatonin protects the body from several kinds of stress damage, stress diminishes melatonin production. Reducing stress will help preserve optimal melatonin levels. In one study, meditating women had higher levels of melatonin than those who did not meditate. On the other hand, when stress is unavoidable, melatonin supplements may help minimize damage.

Class	Example
Nonsteroidal anti-inflammatory drugs (NSAIDS)	aspirin, ibuprofen, indomethacin
Beta-blockers (used in hypertension and heart disease)	propranalol, atenolol, metoprolol
Calcium channel blockers (used in hypertension and heart disease)	nifedipine, isradipine, dilitazem, filodipine, nimodipine, nitrendipine
Sympathetic nervous system inhibitors (used in hypertension)	clonidine, reserpine
Tranquilizers	diazepam, flunitrazepam, alprazolam
Other	caffeine, tobacco, nicotine, alcohol

Table 15. Some common substances that may inhibit melatonin production

TAKING MELATONIN SUPPLEMENTS

Melatonin supplements are relatively new and no firm guidelines have been established as of yet. Dr. Russel Reiter, one of the world's leading experts on melatonin research and usage, recommends the following dosages (further information can be found in the book "Melatonin" by Russel J. Reiter and Jo Robinson):

Usage: Unless otherwise specified by a physician, melatonin should only be taken once a day at bedtime (to emulate the body's physiological rhythm). There is a rather large variation in individual responses to oral melatonin. When absorbed from the GI tract, melatonin passes through the liver where some of it is inactivated. For some, the liver inactivates larger proportions of the ingested dosage than in others, so the same oral dose results in different melatonin blood levels among

and therefore, less melatonin may be needed to achieve the same effect.

Most experts agree that for anti-aging purposes, dosages should emulate the average nighttime level of a young adult (about 100-150 picograms of melatonin per milliliter). Some anti-aging doctors and clinics offer tests to measure nighttime melatonin release and can help you tailor the dosage to your needs. If such testing is unavailable, it is prudent to use a small dose of 0.1-0.2 mg. (You may have to divide a larger tablet).

Usage	Dose Range
Anti-aging	0.1 - 3 mg , taken at bedtime
Sleep	0.2 - 10 mg, taken at bedtime
Jet-lag	1 - 10 mg, taken at bedtime, local time
Shift work	1 - 5 mg, taken at the beginning of designated sleep time
Immune stimulation	2 - 20 mg, as recommended by your physician

DHEA

POSSIBLE BENEFITS, SIDE EFFECTS AND GENERAL PRECAUTIONS

Like growth hormone and melatonin, DHEA increases life span and prevents some degenerative-diseases in laboratory animals. Limited human studies indicate that restoring DHEA levels to those of young adults may provide health and longevity benefits, including, but not

adults may provide health and longevity benefits, including, but not limited to, the following (see Chapter 6 for details):

- Improved mood, sense of well-being and, possibly, memory and learning,
- Modest protection from heart disease in men,
- Improved carbohydrate metabolism and increased insulin sensitivity,
- Improved immunity, particularly the effectiveness of vaccination,
- Possibly, stimulation of sex drive in persons with low DHEA levels. The effect appears to be more significant in women.

DHEA appears to be relatively safe, especially at low doses and over the short-term. No long-term studies are presently available. Nonetheless side effects can and do occur. Dr. Shahelian, the author of "DHEA: A Practical Guide," interviewed a large number of researchers and clinicians about the safety of DHEA and lists the following possible side effects of large doses of DHEA:

- acne and excessive oiliness of skin,
- hair growth in women (in unwanted places),
- deepening of voice,
- irritability or mood changes,
- overstimulation or insomnia,
- fatigue or low energy.

Infrequent side effects possibly attributable to DHEA include headaches, aggressiveness and menstrual irregularity.

The side effects of DHEA, except for a deepening of voice in women, are usually reversed quickly when treatment is stopped or dosage is lowered. At 25 mg a day or less, any side effects are rare. However, some unusually sensitive individuals may notice side effects at doses as low as 5 or 10 mg. Others, however, may take 100 or 200

Some scientists speculate that the ability of DHEA to increase the production of male and female sex steroids may promote the growth of sex hormone responsive tumors, such as breast cancer in women and prostate cancer in men. There is no data to either support or deny this possibility.

Taking DHEA supplements

Like melatonin, DHEA is available over-the-counter and is relatively inexpensive. There are no clear guidelines on DHEA dosage and usage. Most experts agree that the goal should be to restore, but not exceed, DHEA levels in young adults. It would be wise to consult a doctor who has experience in DHEA therapy and review your medical history in the light of possible treatment. Once a decision to proceed is made, DHEA levels should be measured before treatment and then adjusted to achieve optimal levels. Most laboratories offer tests for both DHEA and DHEAS (the form of DHEA whose level is more indicative of total DHEA production, see Chapter 7). Although DHEA tends to decline with age, there is significant individual variation. It shouldn't be assumed that any young person would have high DHEA(S) levels and older individual, lower ones.

Unfortunately, there is a poor correlation between the oral dose of DHEA and blood levels. When taken orally and absorbed from the GI tract, most steroidal hormones (including DHEA) are partly metabolized by the liver before being distributed to the rest of the body. Part of the DHEA is converted by the liver to estrogens and androgens. The remainder enters the body's general circulation. How much DHEA finally gets into the bloodstream varies considerably. Begin with low doses of 5-10 mgs a day. Your health care provider may recommend an increase to the dosage by 5-10 mg every week or two until youthful DHEA blood levels or other appropriate effects have been achieved. DHEA usually comes in 25 or 50 mg capsules or tablets, but you can obtain a smaller dose by simply opening the capsule and dividing the content.

Natural DHEA production peaks in the early morning and falls off during the day. Most physicians recommend taking DHEA supplements in the morning to match this natural rhythm. Some doctors suggest taking about 2/3 of the daily dose in the morning and the rest at night.

For more information on DHEA replacement we suggest the book by Dr. Ray Shahelian, "DHEA: A Practical Guide."

Boosting your own DHEA production

Is there a way to boost one's DHEA levels without taking supplements? There are a number of ways to increase your DHEA levels, although to go from "very low" to "perfect" is next to impossible. The best way to keep one's DHEA levels high is by avoiding stress. If possible, lead a more relaxed lifestyle, be in a "good mood", and deal with depression if it comes along. Both DHEA(S) and the key stress hormone, cortisol, are made from the same precursor, pregnenolone. Stress tends to switch the supply of pregnenolone towards the production of cortisol rather than DHEA(S), causing DHEA(S) levels to go down. Hence the fewer stresses, the more DHEA. Regular meditation appears to raise DHEA levels.

As cited earlier, one study demonstrated a dramatic rise in DHEA(S) levels following a treatment with a drug that reduced insulin excess and improved glucose tolerance. Improving carbohydrate tolerance and insulin sensitivity with other methods, such as high-fiber diet and exercise may also raise DHEA levels.

A few vitamin companies promote wild yam supplements as a "natural" form of DHEA or "DHEA precursor" preparations. Their advertising usually implies that plant steroids found in wild yam, such as diosgenin, can be converted to DHEA by the body. These supplements are supposedly even better than actual DHEA, simply because the body will convert into DHEA only as much plant precursors as it body will convert into DHEA only as much plant precursors as it needs.

Diosgenin and related sterols can be converted into DHEA in the laboratory through a series of chemical reactions. There is no evidence whatsoever that such conversion occurs in humans. In all likelihood, wild yam has no effect on the levels of DHEA or DHEAS.

CHAPTER 26

THE GREATEST MASS MURDERER IN HISTORY

Hitler slaughtered more than six million Jews. Stalin butchered staggering numbers of people. But one killer has claimed more lives than all of the monsters and mass-murderers in history combined. Every year, this killer accounts for one third of all deaths in the civilized world. It goes by many names: **atherosclerosis**, a.k.a., arterial sclerosis, heart disease and stroke.

Atherosclerosis is the formation of fatty, fibrous plaques (tumor-like structures) in arterial walls, which can eventually obstruct blood flow completely. Atherosclerosis can reduce or cut blood supply to any organ and damage or ultimately destroy it. The deadliest complications of atherosclerosis are heart disease and stroke. Atherosclerosis is also a common cause of impotence and kidney insufficiency and a host of other conditions leading to limb amputation. What makes atherosclerosis so deadly is that it often has no symptoms until it reaches a very advanced stage. The first symptom of atherosclerosis is often the last - a fatal heart attack or a stroke. Needless to say, just because a person doesn't show any cardiovascular irregularities, they should still take every measure possible to prevent the onset of this modern day plague.

Like all degenerative-diseases, the risk of atherosclerosis increases dramatically with age. Shifts in the body's premenopausal metabolism and hormonal balance contribute to its development. (Women are less likely to develop atherosclerosis than men because of the protective effect of estrogens).

MAJOR RISK FACTORS FOR ATHEROSCLEROSIS

- High LDL cholesterol
- Males 45 years or older
- Females 55 years or older or with premature menopause and not on estrogen replacement
- Hypertension
- High homocysteine
- Low HDL cholesterol
- Smoking
- Diabetes or poor carbohydrate tolerance
- Family history of early heart disease

Development of atherosclerotic plaque is a complex process influenced by several factors. The popular view is that it begins with some form of micro-injury to the internal lining of blood vessels (endothelium); this injury can be produced by blood flow, especially if there's excessive pressure within the vessel. This is why plaque is more likely to develop where larger arteries branch into smaller ones and why hypertension is a risk factor for atherosclerosis. Cardiovascular injuries change the properties of blood vessel lining in such a way that cholesterol-rich lipids circulating in the bloodstream accumulate in the injured area which causes the formation of a soft fatty streak. Fatty streaks are the first sign of atherosclerosis and may develop as early as childhood. As the damage increases, monocytes (a type of immune cells) and platelets (cells involved in blood clotting) adhere to the damaged area and promote growth and hardening of plaque. In addition, they release special molecules (growth factors) which stimulate the growth of smooth vascular muscle, causing more narrowing of the vessel. In the final stage, a hard fibrous crust consisting of collagen, elastin, glycosaminoglycan and calcium deposits forms over the plaque. Cholesterol and fat continue to accumulate until the artery is entirely blocked. Plaque may block up to 90% of the artery until noticeable symptoms appear.

Atherosclerotic plaque may grow at different rates or even regress depending on several key factors:

Lipid profile Blood carries lipids (cholesterol and fat) packed in sphere-shaped particles called lipoproteins. Two kinds of lipoproteins have an important role in the development of atherosclerosis, low-density lipoproteins (LDL) and high-density lipoproteins (HDL). The main role of LDL is to transport cholesterol to the tissues (cholesterol is required by cells for building membranes). Unfortunately, atherosclerotic plaques contributing to their growth can also capture LDL. HDL, on the other hand, removes excess cholesterol from tissues and transports it to the liver for recycling. Thus the more LDL ("bad cholesterol") and less HDL ("good cholesterol") a person has, the more quickly plaque will grow and vice versa. Indeed, LDL levels as well as LDL/HDL ratio are much better indicators of the potential of heart disease than total cholesterol by itself.

According to the American Heart Association, the desirable level for LDL is 130 mg/dl or less (100 mg/dl or less for people with existing heart disease), and for total cholesterol - 200 mg/dl or less.

Free radicals The rate at which LDL is gobbled up by plaque depends not only on LDL content in the bloodstream, but also how "sticky" the LDL are. Evidence indicates that free radical damage makes LDL stickier and therefore more likely to cause atherosclerosis. Whatever promotes free radical formation, such as smoking, stress or some nutrient deficiencies (particularly deficiencies of vitamins A, C, E, selenium, zinc and copper), tends to promote atherosclerosis. On the other hand, antioxidants may help slow it down.

Platelets aggregation Platelets are small cells that participate in clot formation during injury. They clump together and form a clot that blocks the outflow of blood from the wound. If we didn't have platelets we would literally bleed to death. But there is a price to pay. Sometimes platelets may form small clots even when there is no injury or even when the injury is microscopic, like a tiny lesion in the vascular lining. These small clots can become embedded in the atherosclerotic plaque causing it to grow. The excessive tendency of platelets to "congregate" promotes atherosclerosis. Conversely, reducing their mutual attraction, does the opposite. Aspirin, for instance, can reduce platelet aggregation, which is the reason why it is often prescribed to those at risk of a heart attack. Some nutrients, such as omega-3 fatty acids, can do the same thing, but with less risk of side effects.

Homocysteine During protein breakdown, the amino acid methionine is converted to its derivative, homocysteine. At high levels, homocysteine has the potential to damage the cells of the vascular lining. Normally, the level of homocysteine is low and relatively harmless because it is quickly transformed into another non-toxic derivative. However, in those who are deficient in folic acid and vitamin B6, the conversion of homocysteine is slower and its levels are high. Evidence strongly suggests that this may contribute to atherosclerosis.

IMPAIRED CARBOHYDRATE TOLERANCE AND DIABETES Aging is associated with a tendency toward impaired carbohydrate tolerance and increased risk of diabetes. Elevated blood glucose seen in these conditions contributes to atherosclerosis in many ways. In particular, glucose promotes cross-linking of arterial walls making them less elastic and more susceptible to injury. As arteries stiffen, blood pressure rises, further worsening atherosclerosis. Also, individuals with early stages of type II diabetes and impaired carbohydrate tolerance tend to have elevated insulin levels, which is an important contributor to elevation of LDL and rise in blood pressure.

WHAT TO DO ABOUT ATHEROSCLEROSIS

It is more evident with atherosclerosis than other age-related diseases that an ounce of prevention is worth a pound of cure. Especially when you consider that the first sign of any problem may result in your funeral. While the progression of atherosclerosis can be stopped or even partially reversed, some of the damage after a heart attack or stroke is usually irreversible and can impair the quality of life for the rest of one's days. For anyone concerned with life extension or simply good quality of life, reasonable steps to prevent atherosclerosis are not elective; they're mandatory.

Like other typical age-related disease, many of the life extension measures discussed here will help forestall it to some degree. However, due to the seriousness of its nature, we feel compelled to discuss specific measures to combat atherosclerosis.

DIET: FAT, CHOLESTEROL, SUGAR, FIBER, AND CALORIES

There are three types of fat in most diets: saturated, monounsaturated and polyunsaturated. Today, there is abundant evidence that saturated fat promotes atherosclerosis. The link between saturated fat and atherosclerosis was first suspected when there was a marked decline in mortality from coronary heart disease during the Great Depression and World War II.

In those days people consumed less milk, butter, cheese and eggs. Therefore, they consumed less saturated fat. It was also noted that societies with low consumption of animal fat, a main source of saturated fat, had a substantially lower mortality rate resulting from heart disease. Some critics argued that differences in heart disease incidence between nations might be due to the differences in genetic predisposition of their populations. This does not appear to be true. For instance, Japanese immigrants in the U.S. who have adopted a typical American diet have significantly higher incidence of heart diseases than those who maintain a typical Japanese diet.

An enormous body of experimental research and clinical studies also demonstrates that saturated fat increases LDL cholesterol levels and promotes atherosclerosis. As a first step to reduce elevated LDL, most experts recommend reducing total fat consumption to 30% of total calories and saturated fat no more than 10%. If LDL does not return to the normal range, saturated fat should be further reduced to less than 7% of total calories.

Avoiding excessive amounts of saturated fat is a smart and healthy decision. Some people simply switch from butter to margarine.

Margarine, which is made from the oil of various plants usually has much less saturated fat than butter. However, the chemical process used in producing margarine leads to the formation of so-called trans-monounsaturated fat which is equally bad or worse than saturated fat. Unsaturated fatty acids have two alternative structural forms; *cis* and *trans*. Essentially all unsaturated fat in nature is found in cis form. However, the process of oil hydrogenation used to produce margarine yields significant amount of *trans*-monounsaturated fat, which is at least as atherogenic as saturated fat. It is recommended to use margarine with little or no trans fat. If the information about trans fat content is missing on the label, call the manufacturer. Solid margarine brands tend to have more *trans* fat. Trans fat can also be hidden in processed foods. If the list of ingredients include the term "vegetable shortening" (which is essentially low quality margarine), be aware that the product is likely to have *trans* fat in it.

Some people go to extremes using large amount of polyunsaturated fat in an attempt to avoid saturated and trans fat. This indeed lowers LDL and may even raise HDL (assuming total calories are not in excess). However, polyunsaturated fat, especially when cooked or exposed to air for prolonged periods, increases free radical damage. This has a host of negative effects including damage to arteries. Yet another fallacy is to embark on a low fat diet which may lead to the subclinical deficiency of essential fatty acids.

Overall, monounsaturated fat appears to be the healthiest and should constitute the largest share of your total fat consumption. The best sources of monounsaturated fats are **olive** and **canola oil.**

Simply reducing saturated fat by itself is not nearly enough. Excess calories are just as bad, or perhaps worse, than saturated fat. The body stores calories it can't use as fat, no matter what the source. Even if none of your excess calories come from fat, the body will convert it to fat for storage - mostly saturated fat. And before this fat gets tucked away in your fat tissue, it will circulate in your blood and promote atherosclerosis. The most straightforward way to ensure that you do not consume excess calories is to get as close as possible to your optimal weight and stay there. Bouncing up and down the scale can be extremely hazardous to your health.

Most people are afraid of cholesterol-rich foods, assuming the more cholesterol consumed, the higher the blood cholesterol. This may sound logical, but it really isn't. Most of the cholesterol that circulates in the blood is produced in the body and only a relatively small portion comes from food. Furthermore, dietary cholesterol inhibits the production of cholesterol by the liver, so the net amount of cholesterol in the bloodstream is almost the same for a relatively wide range of dietary foods. However, very large amounts of cholesterol in your diet (such as eating several eggs every day) may upset this equilibrium and push your cholesterol levels up. Also, in a minority of people, the inhibition of cholesterol synthesis by dietary cholesterol is not very efficient, so that even a moderately high intake may adversely affect your lipid profile.

Does this mean that people shouldn't reduce their cholesterol intake? In theory, probably so. In practice, probably not. Cholesterol is found exclusively in animal products such as meat, whole milk, dairy and eggs. Cholesterol-rich foods are also rich in saturated fat and calories so when you cut your cholesterol intake you automatically cut your saturated fat and caloric intake. The last is far more important in reducing your LDL cholesterol. So we indeed should avoid cholesterol-rich foods, not to decrease cholesterol, but to cut down on saturated fat and calories.

Excessive consumption of simple carbohydrates, such as sugar or honey is discouraged because they tend to elevate the levels of insulin which in turn promotes atherosclerosis. Fructose, a part of sucrose (table sugar) and a major ingredient in honey, seems to have additional atherogenic effect. Furthermore, simple sugars are the generally the major source of excess calories.

Fiber in the diet helps prevent atherosclerosis in several important ways. Firstly, soluble fiber, found in foods like oats or apples, can help lower cholesterol by binding bile acids and increasing their excretion. Bile acids are derived from cholesterol by the body, so the more that is excreted, the more cholesterol has to be diverted for the synthesis of new bile acids. The net result is a decrease in cholesterol levels.

	Step 1	Step 2
Energy	Adequate to achieve and maintain optimal weight	Adequate to achieve and maintain optimal weight
Total fat*	<30%	<30%
Saturated fat*	8-10%	<7%
Polyunsaturated fat*	Up to 10%	Up to 10%
Monounsaturated fat*	10-15%	10-15%
Cholesterol	<300 mg/day	<200 mg/day

* Expressed as percentage of total calories in the diet

Table 16. Diet characteristics to help reduce LDL cholesterol. Based on data from N. E. Ernst and co-authors. The national cholesterol education program for dietetic practitioners from the Adult Treatment Panel Recommendations. Journal of American Dietetic Association 88 (1988): 1401-1411.

Secondly, high fiber foods are usually low in fat and calories. Finally, fiber slows down the absorption of glucose from the GI tract, to result in lower blood glucose and insulin levels, which also helps prevent atherosclerosis.

<u>Omega-3 fatty acids</u>: Omega-3 fatty acids are unsaturated fatty acids found in fish oil. They have a wide array of effects on the body because they change the fluidity of cellular membranes. Most importantly, they serve as precursors to prostaglandins. They are the mediators of many types of interactions between cells. Consuming omega-3 fatty acids changes the relative abundance of various prostaglandins in the body. Among other things, omega-3 fatty acids help prevent atherosclerosis by reducing clot formation and blood pressure. The best way to consume omega-3 fat is to have fish at least 2-4 times a week. Cold water fish, such as **salmon** or **cod**, are the best source of omega-

3 fatty acids. Cook fish without extensive frying because omega-3 fat is very susceptible to oxidation.

Antioxidants Various antioxidants, such as vitamins C, E, lipoic acid and polyphenols, prevent or slow down the oxidation of LDL particles. This makes LDL particles less sticky and thus retards the growth of atherosclerotic plaques. Evidence indicated that antioxidant rich foods or supplements reduce the risk of atherosclerosis.

Folic acid, Vitamin B6 and B12 Deficiencies of folic acid, vitamin B6 and possibly B12 may promote atherosclerosis by increasing the levels of homocysteine. The best dietary sources of folic acid are uncooked green leafy vegetables. Aspirin, antacids and oral contraceptives may interact with folic acid adding to the risk of deficiency. Vitamin B12 is present mainly in foods of animal origin. Vitamin B6 is widely distributed among foods, but can be destroyed by prolonged cooking. A healthy person consuming a balanced diet that includes fresh fruits and vegetables is usually not at risk for deficiency of any of these vitamins. Otherwise, one should take a supplement that includes folate, B6 and B12 (100 percent RDA). Larger doses do not add extra protection against atherosclerosis.

Soy protein Several recent studies have demonstrated that consuming about 25-50 gms of soy protein a day can substantially lower LDL and total cholesterol. In these studies, soy protein was not just a supplement to regular diet but replaced some of the animal protein consumed by the subjects. Some researchers believe that much of the effect may not be due to soy protein itself but rather phytoestrogens, estrogen-like compounds present in soy. Whatever the real cause, consuming a lot of soy products may improve your lipid profile. However, for most people raised in Western culture, working large amounts of soy in one's diet is a considerable challenge.

Exercise Exercise raises HDL "good cholesterol" and helps burn calories. It is helpful in preventing atherosclerosis but clearly insufficient by itself.

Stress reduction Stress promotes atherosclerosis in many ways: by elevating blood sugar, by rising blood pressure, by increasing free radical formation. Stress reduction is at least as important for preventing atherosclerosis as any of the measures discussed above. It was found that Siberian Ginseng, an adaptogen that reduces stress response and counteracts stress-related damage, is very effective in preventing and treating atherosclerosis and its complications.

CHAPTER 27

THE CENTER OF OUR UNIVERSE: THE BRAIN

Its chemical content is worth no more than $30, yet its value is beyond measure. It is without doubt the most complicated mechanism on earth - far more complex than the most sophisticated supercomputer ever built. Without it, life as we know it would cease to exist. It is at the very core of our lives. It is the human brain.

A properly functioning brain makes all other faculties and possessions valuable. Some people say that they would be willing to trade brain power for physical fitness or good looks. However, the brain represents more than intellect. It is our memories, emotions, motor coordination, senses, as well as self-awareness, identity and personality. Our brains determine most of who we are, how we interact with the world and what we are capable of achieving.

Not surprisingly, deterioration of various aspects of the brain function is the most devastating consequence of the aging process. While aging of other organs destroys our bodies, aging of the brain destroys our will, our desires - the very core of who we are. You'd be hard pressed to find anyone who would want to outlive their psychological identity or the ability to think and remember.

Several interrelated processes contribute to functional deterioration of the brain with age:

Death of neurons Neurons may die from damage inflicted by free radicals, stress hormones, toxins, blockage of blood flow or other causes.

Accumulation of age pigments Lipofuscin and other age pigments accumulate in neurons, congesting intracellular flow and impairing function.

Decline in energy production Neurons gradually "burn" their power stations, mitochondria, which lose the ability to produce enough energy (ATP) for normal function.

Reduced blood supply Atherosclerosis and hypertension damage arteries and capillaries supply blood to the brain. Reduced blood supply means reduced brain activity and diminished capacity to withstand stress.

Declining levels of neurotransmitters Our brain function depends on the ability of neurons to communicate efficiently. Reduced functional capacity of neurons leads to their decreased ability to produce the neurotransmitters needed for communication. As a result, neurons with preserved function do not get enough stimulation from their partners, which leads to further functional decline.

Aging of the brain increases the risk of two major types of disorders: mood disorders, such as depression and cognitive disorders, such as Alzheimer's disease, dementia and memory loss. It appears that nutritional supplements significantly effect the rate at which the brain ages. Furthermore, slowing down brain aging also seems to decelerate the aging of the body.

Mental capacity

Mental capacity is a broad term which includes cognitive ability, memory, communication skills and the ability to meet the mental requirements of daily life. While some loss of mental capacity with age is inevitable, the rate may vary dramatically due to great variations in the rate of aging mechanisms. A profound loss of mental capacity is usually referred to as dementia. It was estimated that about 15% - 20% of the elderly in America have some form of dementia. Alzheimer's disease is responsible for half of all cases of dementia, while the rest are due to a wide variety of causes including Parkinson's disease, stroke, B vitamin deficiency, hypothyroidism and others.

Alzheimer's disease is characterized by the degeneration of neurons in the brain areas responsible for mental functions. The most common physiological findings in Alzheimer's disease are low levels of acetylcholine (a neurotransmitter especially important for mental capacity), reduced brain circulation, and increased production of free radical and low free radical defenses. Countering these factors delays and sometimes reverses Alzheimer's disease and generally helps preserve mental capacity.

FOOD SUPPLEMENTS THAT HELP PRESERVE OR IMPROVE MENTAL CAPACITY

DMAE

DMAE (dymethylaminoethyl) is a nutrient found in small amounts in fish. It has a variety of beneficial effects on mental capacity. It improves memory, alertness, concentration, chronic fatigue and mild depression. In one study it was even found to improve I.Q. Deanol, a drug similar in structure and action to DMAE, has been successfully used to treat learning and behavioral problems such as attention deficit disorder and hyperkinesia. An intriguing side effect of DMAE in some patients is lucid dreaming, a state in which a person is aware that they are dreaming. Most people consider lucid dreaming a highly enjoyable and interesting experience. In some, but not all rodent studies, DMAE was found to increase life span by up to 30%.

DMAE appears to exert its action by elevating brain levels of acetylcholine, a neurotransmitter involved in a variety of mental functions. As we mentioned, Alzheimer's disease and some other types of dementia are associated with low levels of acetylcholine in the brain.

Several animal studies have shown that DMAE reduces the accumulation of the age pigment lipofuscin in the brain. Evidence indicates that this effect may be due to the ability of DMAE to stimulate antioxidant enzymes and inhibit cross-linking. Thus, DMAE appears not only to stimulate mental functions but actually slows down brain aging.

DMAE is available as a nutrient supplement. Usual doses are between 500 and 1000 mg a day. However, one should start with a low dose of 50 or 100 mg a day and build up gradually. DMAE is often sold as DMAE bitartrate which contains only a percentage of DMAE. If using DMAE bitartrate, the dosages should be calculated according to the content of pure DMAE. It may take 2-4 weeks to feel the full effects of DMAE.

CAUTION: People with epilepsy or manic depressive disorders should not use DMAE. High doses of DMAE can produce insomnia, headaches and muscle tenderness. Side effects usually disappear when the dose is lowered. If you are taking any medications, especially cholinergics, consult your doctor before using DMAE.

GINKGO BILOBA

Ginkgo biloba is one of the oldest tree species on Earth. It has been widely used in traditional Chinese medicine for such diverse maladies as circulation problems, impaired hearing, sexual dysfunction and memory loss.

In recent decades, the biological effects of Ginkgo biloba extract have been extensively studied in both animals and humans. It was shown that Ginkgo biloba extract is beneficial in a wide variety of central nervous system disorders, including: dementia, memory loss, decreased concentration and cognitive ability, impaired vision, hearing loss, vertigo, and many other maladies. In healthy individuals, Ginkgo biloba extract improves concentration, alertness and short-term memory. Today, Ginkgo biloba extract is one of the most prescribed medications in Europe for age-related disorders of mental capacity.

The remarkable benefits of Ginkgo biloba extract provide the central nervous system are due to the synergy of several effects. First, it enhances brain circulation, improving the delivery of oxygen and nutrients to neurons. Second, it protects neurons from free radical damage - the brain is especially vulnerable to free radicals because of the high content of lipids which are easy targets for oxidation. Finally, Ginkgo biloba inhibits the aggregation of clot-forming cells, which reduces the formation of new blood clots and may even unclog partially occluded arteries.

The recommended dose of Ginkgo biloba extract is 40 mg 3 times a day. Usually, a standardized extract containing 24% of ginkgo heterosides is used. For less concentrated extracts, the dose should be correspondingly higher. Adverse reactions are rare and usually mild, and include gastrointestinal upset and headaches.

Choline

Choline is a precursor used by the body to synthesize acetylcholine, one of the key neurotransmitters in higher mental functions. Choline supplementation increases brain levels of acetylcholine, and is shown to improve memory and learning in normal subjects. Unfortunately, choline is rarely effective in patients with Alzheimer's disease because they are usually deficient in the enzyme that synthesizes acetylcholine from choline. Usual doses of choline are 1-3 gms a day.

Antioxidants

The brain requires more reliable antioxidant protection than any other organ in the body. While it constitutes only about 2% of body mass, the brain burns about 20% of all calories. Brain tissue is bombarded by up to 10 times as many free radicals than most other tissues. Besides, the brain is rich in lipids that are easily damaged by free radicals. To protect themselves, brain cells produce large amounts of antioxidant enzymes. However, even a slight weakening of antioxidant defenses due to stress, disease, nutrient deficiency or age-related physiological changes (e.g. decline in melatonin production or reduced circulation) can upset this delicate balance and lead to significant free radical damage. Antioxidant supplements may help reduce free radical damage to the brain. Of particular importance for neuroprotection are lipid soluble antioxidants such as vitamin E, lipoic acid and melatonin.

DEPRESSION

As we discussed earlier, depression is one of the most common consequences of the age-related decline in brain function and specifically, the decline in the levels of neurotransmitters. While depression is often a consequence of aging, it is also a factor in the acceleration of the aging process. Depression contributes to aging by causing excessive stress, suppressing the immune system, and possibly speeding up the central aging clock. One of the most consistent psychological findings in the study of centenarians is positive mental attitude, emotional stability and good coping ability, the opposites of depression. Relieving depression is an important part of anti-aging strategy. Not merely because it helps slow down some of the mechanisms of aging, but also because depression reduces a person's motivation for positive action.

The biochemical basis of depression is a decrease in the levels of neurotransmitters in the brain. Most modern antidepressant drugs work by raising the levels of neurotransmitters, particularly serotonin and norepinephrine. Side effects are common, and include sedation, constipation, nausea, dry mouth, GI distress, lightheadedness, impotence and others. For that reason, drug treatment is usually reserved for clinically significant depression. A number of nutrients and food supplements have been found to produce a marked antidepressant effect with far fewer side effects. This may be especially useful by people with subclinical depression which is extremely common but often goes unnoticed and untreated. Keep in mind that serious depression requires professional treatment by a mental health professional.

Depression and nutrient deficiencies

Before embarking on any antidepressant therapy, one should consider a possibility that depression may be secondary to some other problem. In particular, a deficiency of some nutrients is a relatively common cause of depression.

Vitamin B12

Depression is one of many possible symptoms of vitamin B12 deficiency. Others include psychosis, irritability, confusion, memory loss, nerve damage and anemia. However, in mild B12 deficiency, depression may be the only symptom. It is not entirely clear why B12 deficiency causes depression and other mental disorders. B12 is required for the synthesis of S-adenosylmethionine (SAM) from methionine. Whereas SAM has a role in the synthesis of some neurotransmitters, particularly serotonin, it is generally believed that B12 deficiency leads to depression by disturbing neurotransmitter synthesis via this pathway.

B12 is unique among vitamins in that it is found almost exclusively in foods of animal origin such as meat, poultry, fish, eggs and dairy products. Contrary to popular belief, no active form of B12 is found in algae such as spirulina or fermented soy products. This means that strict vegetarians are at risk of vitamin B12 deficiency. Since the liver stores large amounts of B12, it takes from several months to several years for an overt deficiency to develop. However, depression may develop long before other symptoms. Nutritionists generally recommend that strict vegetarians (vegans) take B12 supplements.

Healthy young and middle-aged people consuming a balanced non-vegetarian diet are usually not at risk for vitamin B12 deficiency. The absorption of vitamin B12 from food requires an intrinsic factor, a protein produced by the stomach. Some elderly do not produce enough intrinsic factor due to the atrophy of stomach glands, common in advanced age. This may lead to B12 deficiency. Another possible, if rare cause of B12 deficiency is pernicious anemia, a condition seen in all ages in which the stomach produces no acid. Vitamin B12 status is usually assessed by measuring its plasma levels.

RDA for B12 is 2 ml a day that is usually sufficient to prevent deficiency in a healthy vegatarian. However, oral administration is often ineffective in people with poor B12 absorption. Until recently, injections were the only alternative, but effective intranasal preparations are now also available. Occasionally, depressed individuals with apparently normal B12 blood levels respond to large doses of B12 (250 - 1,000 mg a day).

Folate

A deficiency in folate is a relatively common finding in depression. It is estimated that about 30% of psychiatric patients are folate-deficient. In one study, 2 out of 3 geriatric patients admitted to a psychiatric ward were folate-deficient. Other symptoms of folate deficiency include mental confusion, anemia, heartburn, diarrhea, malabsorption, and decreased immunity. Like B12, folate is involved in the synthesis of SAM. Folate and B12 deficiency are likely to cause depression through the same mechanism.

Vegetables are the most abundant sources of folate, particularly green leafy vegetables and beans. The only food from animal source rich in folate is liver. Folate can be destroyed during cooking and prolonged storage. The best way to obtain enough folate from the diet is to eat generous amounts of fresh or slightly cooked vegetables. Diets lacking vegetables and fruit put you at risk for folate deficiency. Long-term use of aspirin and antacids may cause folate deficiency by interfering with the absorption of folate. Oral contraceptives and smoking may also impair folate status. Folate status is assessed by a plasma folate test or by a red blood cell folate test which is far more accurate.

RDA for folate is 180 mg a day for women and 200 mg for men. Clinically proven deficiency is usually treated with 1,000 mg of folate per day. To correct a possible deficiency, experts usually recommend 400 mg a day supplements. In some cases, folate supplementation may result in a complete resolution of the symptoms of depression, or at least enhance the effectiveness of other measures.

Niacin

Niacin (nicotinic acid) is unique among vitamins in that it can be synthesized in the body from an amino acid, tryptophan. The body uses about 60 mg of tryptophan to produce 1mg of niacin. While niacin deficiency in developed countries is unlikely (unless you are a popcorn-and-soda junkie), low niacin intake will divert significant amounts of tryptophan to the synthesis of niacin. This leaves less tryptophan for its other uses which includes the synthesis of serotonin. Supplementing niacin is sometimes helpful as an adjunct measure in the treatment of depression because it may help increase serotonin synthesis. RDA for niacin is 15 mg for women and 19 mg for men.

Depression and food supplements

5-hydroxytryptophan

5-hydroxytryptophan (5-THP) is very much like Prozac - only better! This is not a particularly scientific statement, but rather it is actually an accurate one. Like Prozac, 5-HTP relieves depression by raising brain levels of serotonin. The effectiveness of 5-HTP and Prozac in depression is probably about the same, but 5-HTP has fewer side-effects. This makes it an overall better form of treatment.

The difference between 5-HTP and Prozac is the way in which they achieve higher serotonin levels. Prozac is a drug belonging to a class of selective serotonin uptake inhibitors (SSRI). It acts by blocking the reuptake of serotonin by neurons after the impulse has been transmitted. As a result, more serotonin remains active in the synaptic cleft, leading to greater activity of serotoninergic neurons (the neurons that use serotonin as a main neurotransmitter).

5-HTP, on the other hand, is a nutrient and a metabolite. The body creates serotonin from the amino acid tryptophan derived from proteins in food. First, tryptophan is converted to 5-HTP which is then converted to serotonin. Thus 5-HTP is an immediate precursor of serotonin. Tryptophan was used to treat depression for decades. In the Eighties, there were several cases of serious side effects linked to the use of tryptophan supplements which resulted in an FDA ban. The problem was traced to a single contaminated batch allegedly produced by a new, untested method. Nonetheless, the FDA has not lifted its ban. As opposed to tryptophan, 5-HTP is available over-the-counter and appears to be more effective than tryptophan. This is understandable. 5-HTP is only one metabolic step removed from serotonin.

Several studies compared the effectiveness of 5-HTP to commonly used antidepressants. 5-HTP was found to be at least as effective as imipramine, a common tricyclic antidepressant, or fluvoxamine, an SSRI similar to Prozac. In both of these studies, 5-HTP was better tolerated than the antidepressant. Other studies indicate that 5-HTP may be useful in other disorders associated with serotonin deficiency and commonly treated with SSRI, such as: anxiety, insomnia, aggressiveness, agitation, obsessive compulsive behavior and migraines. 5-HTP also appears to reduce appetite and may be useful along with a healthy diet in a weight reduction program.

The dosage of 5-HTP used in most clinical studies was 300 mg a day (taken as 100 mg three 3 times a day); Doses as low as 50 or 100 mg a day may be effective for mild depression. A physician should determine the right dosage.

Vitamin B6

Vitamin B6 is a co-factor in the synthesis of serotonin from 5-HTP. RDA for B6 is 1.6 mg for women and 2 mg for men. B6 deficiency is very rare since this vitamin is found in a wide variety of foods. Supplemental B6 was shown to increase serotonin synthesis in animals. B6 supplements should be most effective when used in combination with 5-HTP. A dose of 10-20 mg a day of B6 is usually recommended. Keep in mind that B6 has a potential for toxicity. High doses (hundreds of milligrams) of B6 taken for extended periods have been linked to cases of irreversible nerve damage.

DL-PHENYLALANINE

DL-phenylalanine is an equal mixture of D and L isoforms of the amino acid phenylalanine. L-phenylalanine is a precursor of the neurotransmitters norepinephrine and dopamine, and may raise the brain levels of these neurotransmitters facilitating the relief of depression. D-phenylalanine is an inhibitor of the enzyme enkephalinase. This enzyme precipitates the degradation of enkephalins, physiologically produced morphine-like compounds that act as anti-stress agents and painkillers. Also, phenylalanine can be converted in the body to phenylethylamine, a substance with both stimulant and antidepressant properties. Apparently the combination of the above effects are responsible for the marked antidepressant activity of DL-phenylalanine, which has been demonstrated in several clinical trials. In one study, DL-phenylalanine was found to be as effective as the prescription antidepressant imipramine but with fewer side effects. In most studies, DL-phenylalanine was used at doses from 200 to 500 mg a day. The right dosage is best determined by a physician.

ST. JOHN'S WORT

St. John's Wort (*Hypericum perforatum*) is an herb with a long history in the treatment of depression and anxiety. Extracts from St. John's Wort appear to exert an antidepressant action via weak inhibition of the enzyme monoamine oxidase, as well a number of other effects on the central nervous system.

Compared to most other medicinal herbs, St. John's Wort has been thoroughly researched. It was found that much of its action was due to the substance named hypericin. Most extracts used in clinical studies were standardized for their hypericin content. A large number of well-conducted clinical trials demonstrated the effectiveness of hypericin in depression and anxiety.

German researchers performed the meta-analysis (a type of statistical analysis which compares and combines the results of several different studies) of 23 clinical trials of St. John's Wort extracts. The studies involved a total of 1,757 patients with mild or moderate depressive disorders and the analysis confirmed the efficiency of St. John's Wort in the treatment of depression. Evidence indicates that it was similar in effectiveness to standard antidepressants such as imipramine. St. John's Wort, however, was much better tolerated than standard antidepressants. Side effects occurred in 52.8% of patients treated with antidepressants, but only in 19.8% of patients treated with St. John's Wort extracts. The doses of St. John's Wort extracts used in most studies supplied from 2 to 2.7 mg of hypericin a day. However, some side effects are possible at these or even lower doses. A physician should supervise treatment with St. John's Wort.

CHAPTER 28

ADAPTOGENS: A BETTER WAY OF DEALING WITH STRESS

Adaptogens are arguably one of the most effective weapons in combating various types of stress. As one gathers from the name, adaptogens are substances, most often of plant origin, that promote a successful adaptation to all sorts of challenges. The term **adaptogen** was coined in the late Forties by a Russian researcher, Dr. N. Lazerev, who found that some substances could enhance the resistance of test subjects to various adverse situations. Another Russian researcher, Dr. I. Brekhman, further developed the concept of adaptogens as substances that fulfill the following criteria:

- Adaptogens enhance resistance to a wide variety of damaging or stressful factors, such as: physical or mental overexertion or trauma, cold, heat, radiation, toxic chemicals, etc. As a result, the body can withstand all kinds of stresses longer and with less damage.
- Adaptogens tend to normalize physiological parameters, whether there is either a deficiency or excess. For instance, many adaptogens can both reduce high blood pressure and raise low blood pressure.
- Adaptogens are non-toxic and produce little or no side effects in a wide range of doses.
- The substances that fulfill all of the above criteria do exist. Some, like ginseng, have been used for centuries. Most adaptogens have some additional capacities such as cognitive enhancement, stimulation of the immune function and others.

Much of adaptogen research was done in the USSR between 1940 and 1980, behind the Iron Curtain. In fact, Soviet scientists performed thousands of adaptogens studies documenting their numerous benefits. The few Western studies that were done corroborate the Soviet data, especially in regard to Siberian Ginseng.

As it turns out, adaptogens have great value not only in stressful situations, but also in dealing with a variety of diseases from nervous system disorders to cancer. Physicians incorporated adaptogens in numerous therapies because of their ability to enhance the effectiveness of other agents and speed recovery in a wide variety of diseases. However, the most appropriate use of adaptogens is in aging and age-related diseases.

Firstly, the loss of adaptability is one of the most intrinsic features of aging. In older people, even a moderate extra burden on the system may cause failure as a result of diminished reserve capacity. Adaptogens reverse this trend. They restore the body's ability to pull the extra load whenever needed. Secondly, aging is associated with various disturbances of homeostasis, the body's internal balance. Adaptogens tend to push the values of various physiological parameters, such as blood pressure, blood sugar, heart rate and cholesterol levels back into the normal range, thus preventing or reversing many age-related diseases. Finally, aging is associated with an excessive stress response. In particular, older people tend to produce excessive amounts of stress steroids in response to stressors, even at rest, which brings on a host of negative consequences. Many adaptogens work towards optimizing the stress response, making it appropriate for the actual needs of the body.

Young people may also benefit from adaptogens, especially when faced with challenges or during recovery from trauma or illness. In a sense, adaptogens can provide an older individual with the physical and mental capacity of a younger one and can give a younger person almost superhuman endurance.

How and why do adaptogens work? Most drugs are quite different from adaptogens in the sense that they target a specific body system or organ and either suppress or stimulate it. An adaptogen is to a typical drug what a general practitioner is to a specialist. Adaptogens optimize general resistance rather than the specific function of a particular organ.

Our understanding of how adaptogens boost general resistance and an adaptive capacity is incomplete. One important characteristic of many adaptogens is to modify the body's stress response. As you may remember, the stress response consists of three main phases: alarm reaction, resistance phase and exhaustion. Often, the alarm reaction is excessive leaving far too few resources for the next phase. Some adaptogens reduce the intensity of the alarm phase and enhance the body's ability to maintain the resistance phase. This reduces stress-related damage and helps avoid the exhaustion phase.

Another highly important characteristic of many adaptogens is their anabolic activity. In essence, this means that adaptogens stimulate the growth of lean tissue. This effect is the opposite of what happens during stress. Stress is associated with intense catabolism, meaning that the body breaks up its lean tissue for fuel. Under such conditions, repair and regeneration of tissue are impeded. Some adaptogens change the mode of fuel utilization to allow for more fat and less protein to be burnt as fuel. This reduces tissue damage and speeds recovery. In addition, some, but not all adaptogens have antioxidant properties, although most antioxidants are not adaptogens.

While they may have many similarities in terms of their overall effects, individual adaptogens often exert their power at very different levels and sites in the body. Individual adaptogens were shown to work on one or all of the following levels:

<u>Central nervous systems</u> Some adaptogens, such as schizandra, were shown to act mainly on the central nervous system, which in turn leads to metabolic shifts in hormone levels.

<u>Endocrine systems</u> Adaptogens may also act on the endocrine glands. For instance, Siberian Ginseng directly modulates the production of stress steroid by the adrenals.

<u>Cellular level</u> Some adaptogens work primarily on the cellular level. **Leuzea carthamoides**, for example, can stabilize mitochondria during

stress, preserving their ability to convert fuel into the cellular energy carrier, ATP.

Adaptogens are excellent endurance enhancers and anti-stress agents. However, their usefulness goes far beyond that. Adaptogens are used in the treatment of diseases as well as preventing or reversing certain aspects of the aging process.

Indeed, two cardinal features of aging are the loss of adaptability and the loss of resistance to stress. Also, if we consider the physiology of a healthy twenty-five-year-old to be the norm, then even a healthy older person will deviate from the norm. Adaptogens help counter both these trends, which make them one of today's most versatile anti-aging tools.

Common Name	Botanical Name	Plant Part
Ginseng	Panax ginseng	root
Siberian Ginseng	Eleutherococcus Senticosus	root
Ashwaganda, Indian ginseng	Withania Somnifera	root, seeds
Tulsi, Holy Basil	Ocimum Sanctum	leaves
Gold root	Rhodiola Rosea	root, rhizome
Schizandra	Schizandra Chinensis	seeds
Leuzea	Leuzea Carthamoides	root

Table 17. Plants with confirmed adaptogenic potential

GINSENG

Ginseng (*Panax ginseng*) is perhaps the single best know medicinal plant in history. Many of ginseng's benefits come from its ability to act as an adaptogen. According to historical records, ginseng has been employed in Chinese folk medicine for at least 3,000 years, but until recently, ginseng's fame had little factual evidence to support it. Over the past few decades, researchers, mainly in Russia and China, have demonstrated that ginseng is an adaptogen with a variety of positive health effects.

Ginseng is a perennial plant with a simple solitary stem up to 25 " long. Its powers lie in its fleshy taproot. Evidence indicates that most of ginseng's biological activity is due to an unusual group of compounds called ginsenosides whose content in the root ranges from 21 to 28%.

Like a typical adaptogen, ginseng increases both physical and mental stamina as well as resistance to a variety of stressors including toxins, radiation, extreme heat and cold. Ginseng reduces blood sugar levels, improves anemia and normalizes blood pressure. Various neurological and endocrine disturbances are also improved with ginseng administration.

Ginseng engages several important physiological mechanisms in the body. Under stress, it improves the fuel efficiency of energy production in the cells. In rats treated with ginseng and subjected to a two hour swim, the breakdown of such energy carriers as glycogen, ATP and creatine-phosphate was reduced, indicating an improved fuel-efficiency. The accumulation of lactate in the muscle, an indicator of exhaustion, was also decreased. Ginseng also shifts the pattern of fuel utilization in the skeletal muscles and the heart muscle towards preferred use of fatty acids over glucose which helps preserve protein from being broken down to synthesize glucose. The body can produce glucose from protein, but not from fat.

Another extremely important benefit of ginseng is that it raises oxygen consumption, enhancing the ability of muscles to extract oxygen from blood. Interestingly, the net result of the metabolic effects of ginseng is very similar to the physical conditioning produced by regular exercise. In a sense, taking a ginseng supplement may be the closest one can get to a workout while still remaining a "couch potato". Nonetheless, we highly recommend exercise.

GINSENG AND STRESS

The ability of ginseng to protect the body from the destructive power of an excessive stress response was first documented by Dr. I. Brekhman. When rats were subjected to severe stress, such as prolonged immobilization or swimming in cold water, they developed a number of characteristic pathological changes, including: enlargement of adrenal glands, shrinkage of the thymus gland and lymph nodes and peptic ulceration. Brekhman showed that ginseng extract provided a significant degree of protection against all these pathological changes. In addition, ginseng abolished the breakdown of tissue proteins and elevation of blood sugar seen during stress. These effects can, in part, be explained by their ability to reduce the intensity of the stress response and improve the responsiveness of tissues to insulin, usually impaired during stress.

GINSENG AS AN ANTIOXIDANT

Ginseng is a highly effective antioxidant. In one study, the glycosides from ginseng and Siberian Ginseng (*Eleutherococcus senticosus*) were tested for their ability to protect red blood cells from free radical damage. Normally, when red blood cells are exposed to high levels of free radicals, they burst because free radicals damage the membranes, making them leaky and fragile. This phenomenon is called oxidative hemolysis. Even very low levels of the glycosides from both "classic" and

Siberian Ginseng were able to prevent oxidative hemolysis of red blood cells. In addition to acting as an antioxidant, ginseng also boosts the cell's antioxidant capacity, accomplished by stimulating the synthesis of NADH, a key co-enzyme and energy carrier which is also a potent antioxidant.

Ginseng may work even more effectively in combination with other antioxidants. In one study, 40 patients with reduced brain circulation due to atherosclerosis were treated with a standard protocol of vasodilating and tranquilizing drugs. Another twenty patients received additional treatment with antioxidants (vitamins E and C) and ginseng extract. This group had a significantly greater improvement in cerebral circulation and a better lipid profile than the control group.

Usage: The dosage of ginseng commonly used in treatment or prevention is nontoxic and rarely produces side effects.

Possible side effects included excitation, insomnia and elevated blood pressure. High doses (10 times higher than therapeutic doses) may produce severe toxicity. Ginseng is usually not recommended in healthy people under 40. The dosage recommended in middle aged people for disease prevention and general anti-aging action is the amount equivalent to 0.25-0.5 gms of dry root 2 or 3 times daily. Ginseng is usually recommended in 15-20 day cycles with at least a two week break in between cycles.

SIBERIAN GINSENG

Siberian Ginseng (*Eleutherococcus senticosus*) is a distant cousin of ginseng (both are members of *Araliaceae* family). It is less known in the West than ginseng, but oriental healers have used it for thousands of years. Since the fifties, Siberian Ginseng has become the focus of Soviet research into adaptogens. Today, there are literally hundreds of published studies on Siberian Ginseng performed in the former Soviet Union, Japan and Europe. Several international symposia were devoted exclusively to Siberian Ginseng.

Why is there so much interest in this plant? Firstly, Siberian Ginseng is highly effective as an adaptogen. In some ways, it's even more effective than "classic" ginseng. Secondly, it is remarkably safe - even relatively high doses usually produce little or no side effects. This is another advantage over classic ginseng. Thirdly, Siberian Ginseng is more widely distributed in nature and far easier to cultivate than classic ginseng. Last, but certainly not least, Siberian Ginseng is relatively inexpensive.

Siberian Ginseng is a shrub, 5-8 ft. tall with elliptic leaves and light gray or brownish bark. It is found in various regions of the Far East. Most of its biological power comes from a group of compounds called eleutherosides whose content is an indicator of potency of Siberian Ginseng preparations.

As a true adaptogen, Siberian Ginseng provides a veritable smorgasbord of health and anti-aging benefits. It counteracts the negative effects of stress, toxins and pollutants, increases physical and mental work capacity, improves immunity, and helps prevent and reverse many age-related diseases.

The action of Siberian Ginseng on the body involves several mechanisms. Similarly to classic ginseng, it accelerates energy production and improves energy efficiency on a cellular level. This is achieved through stimulation of the key enzymes responsible for the utilization of glucose and also by increasing the use of fat for fuel. Another important action of Siberian Ginseng is to temporarily inhibit the production of stress steroids. This effect is extremely important because it reduces the impact of stress steroids on the body. Finally, Siberian Ginseng reduces free radical damage to cellular structures, especially during stress. The net result of all this is that Siberian Ginseng enables the body to adapt to adversity without generating an intense and destructive stress response.

Siberian ginseng and stress

Many studies have shown Siberian Ginseng to dramatically increase resistance to stress and enhance both mental and physical endurance. In one study, researchers studied the capacity of mice to climb an endless cord until complete exhausted. The animals that received a single dose of Siberian Ginseng extract were able to keep going up to 45% longer (depending on the dose) than control animals. In another intriguing study, researchers studied the ability of Siberian Ginseng to reduce mental stress in rats. In rats, just as in people, overcrowding produces significant psychological stress. When given a choice of drinking water or an alcoholic beverage, rats would consume relatively little alcohol under normal conditions. Under the psychological stress of overcrowding, however, the animals consume much more alcohol. Remarkably, rats who regularly received Siberian Ginseng extract consumed 40% less alcohol under these same conditions.

In animals under severe stress, Siberian Ginseng either markedly reduced or completely eliminated serious signs of stress damage. In particular, it prevented ulceration of the gastro-intestinal tract, hypertrophy and hemorrhages in the adrenal glands and breakdown of lean tissue.

There are also a large number of human studies substantiating the stress-reducing and endurance-enhancing effects of Siberian Ginseng. For instance, Dr. Asano from the University of Tsukuba studied the effects of Siberian Ginseng extract on the work capacity in young male athletes. Two milliliters of extract or placebo were administered twice a day for 8 days prior to the test. Siberian Ginseng increased work capacity by a remarkable 23.3% compared to 7.5% rise due to the placebo. Numerous other studies in such diverse groups as airline dispatchers, athletes, telegraph operators, truck drivers and the general population attest to the benefits of Siberian Ginseng in boosting mental and physical performance and stress resistance. Furthermore, with Siberian Ginseng, recovery after a heavy workload proceeds at a much quicker pace.

Siberian Ginseng Improves Resistance to Toxins, Poisons and Pollutants

Another noteworthy attribute of Siberian Ginseng is the reduction of damage caused by toxic chemicals. In a world filled with pollution, food additives and aggressive drug therapy, Siberian Ginseng is truly an asset.

The anti-toxic qualities of Siberian ginseng cover a wide variety of chemicals, although the magnitude of its effects vary based on particular toxins.

In one study, researchers looked into the protective effect of Siberian Ginseng against tetanus endotoxin (a highly toxic chemical produced by tetanus-causing bacteria *Clostridium tetani*). Two groups of mice were injected with the endotoxin, and one of the groups was given a single dose of Siberian Ginseng extract at the dose of 2.5 mg/kg. After 48 hours, all animals that received endotoxin alone were dead, whereas 70% of those additionally treated with Siberian ginseng were alive. Several studies demonstrated Siberian Ginseng reduced the toxic effects of various insecticides and industrial pollutants.

Siberian Ginseng also reduces toxic side effects of many drugs used in chemotherapy. Thus, it can improve the chances of successful completion of these treatments. In experiments on rats with Walker carcinoma, 30% of animals treated with the chemotherapy drug ethymidin died, but all animals receiving Siberian Ginseng survived.

Siberian Ginseng in Prevention and Treatment of Disease

Siberian Ginseng has proved beneficial over a remarkably wide array of conditions, especially age-related diseases. A partial list includes: atherosclerosis, heart disease, stroke, hypertension, mild forms of diabetes, influenza, anemia and kidney insufficiency. In heart disease patients, Siberian Ginseng was shown to reduce or eliminate symptoms, improve eloctro-cardiogram (in as much as 74% of patients in one study) and reduce risk factors such as high blood cholesterol and triglycerides (in one study a marked drop in cholesterol was observed in 51 of 116 patients). Cancer treatment regimens can also be enhanced by Siberian Ginseng because it: reduces toxicity of chemotherapy and radiation, speeds recovery from surgical stress and reduces the risk of relapses by boosting the immune system.

Referring to the therapeutic potential of Siberian Ginseng, Dr. I. Brekhman, a pioneer of adaptogen research wrote:

> *"Siberian Ginseng is not so much a drug for many diseases but rather a medicine for a wide variety of patients whatever their particular health problems might be. Patients would especially benefit from Siberian Ginseng due to its capacity to enhance general resistance of the body. Siberian Ginseng is not a panacea but almost every patient needs it."*

Siberian Ginseng is a remarkably effective preventive medicine. In 1973-1976, thousands of industrial workers in Russia were given an extract of Siberian Ginseng (2 ml a day for two months each year) as a preventative measure. This relatively modest regimen reduced overall disease incidence by up to 35% compared to control groups. There are indications that more extensive use may reduce morbidity even further.

Even more amazing are the results of a Russian study involving 1,200 truck drivers. The subjects were given Siberian Ginseng extract twice a day with tea for two months annually, in spring and fall, for 7 years. There was a dramatic several-fold decrease in the incidence of heart disease, hypertension and flu (other conditions were not documented in the study). The decrease is especially remarkable considering that the participants of the study were getting older and their risk of hypertension and heart disease was supposed to be increasing. A drawback of this study is that there was no control group receiving placebo. However, this is usually more of a problem in short-term studies that involve relatively few individuals as placebo effects are generally short-lived. Such a dramatic effect lasting over the span of 7 years is extremely unlikely to have been due to a placebo. Also, since the group of truck drivers in the study was so large, a general population of truck drivers of similar age can be considered a crude but acceptable control group.

Siberian Ginseng, glucose tolerance and diabetes

As we discussed earlier, elevated blood glucose is a metabolic shift that significantly contributes to the aging process. Marked elevation of blood glucose indicates diabetes. A mild elevation indicates poor

MORBIDITY RATE						
	Influenza		Hypertensive Disease		Ischemic Heart Disease	
Year	Labor Losses	# of cases	Labor Losses	# of cases	Labor Losses	# of cases
1973	286.2	41.77	170.95	6.58	281.82	6.71
1974	171.5	30.49	45.82	3.2	210.04	5.34
1975	188.26	33.03	23.21	2.57	51.05	1.62
1976	144.26	24.04	23.76	2.67	35.24	1.49
1977	73.73	12.86	18.80	1.16	21.47	1.30
1978	31.82	5.72	20.74	2.08	11.96	1.46
1979	11.32	2.75	5.30	0.45	2.98	0.22

Table 18. Effects of Siberian Ginseng extract on morbidity in 2000 truck drivers during the period 1973-1979 (per 100 working drivers).

carbohydrate tolerance which is less dangerous than diabetes but still contributes to premature aging and disease. Bringing blood glucose to optimal levels is an important part of an anti-aging strategy.

Ginseng is modestly effective in lowering blood glucose, while the effect of Siberian Ginseng is at least twice as strong. Siberian Ginseng is very effective in reversing poor carbohydrate tolerance and sometimes even mild cases of diabetes. It can also be used in conjunction with other anti-diabetic measures.

Siberian ginseng as antioxidant and antimutagen

Under stress, the amount of free radicals in the body increases severalfold. They cause damage to many structures; especially biological membranes containing easily oxidized unsaturated fatty acids. In animal studies, Siberian Ginseng reduced the amount of lipid peroxides (the main products of free radical damage to cellular membranes) in stressed animals to levels seen in controls. Antioxidant action of Siberian Ginseng appears to be indirect. Somehow it stimulates the cell's own free radical scavenging systems.

Siberian Ginseng also counteracts the action of mutagens, the substances that causes damage to DNA and tamper with genetic information. In *Drosophila* fruit flies, Siberian Ginseng reduced the rate of mutations caused by N-nitrosomorpholine, a typical mutagen, by about 50%. Furthermore, it also decreased the rate of spontaneous mutations (i.e. mutations in the absence of external mutagens) and increased life span in fruit flies.

OTHER EFFECTS OF SIBERIAN GINSENG

Research on Siberian Ginseng points to numerous other benefits as well. For instance, in healthy young adults who received a single dose of Siberian Ginseng, visual acuity increased by 30% 8 hours after ingestion. Siberian Ginseng enhanced color perception both in normal and color-blind persons. A single dose of 2 ml of Siberian ginseng extract significantly reduced (as compared to placebo) a number of errors made by telegraph operators.

In a large number of studies, Siberian Ginseng significantly improved many aspects of immunity. In particular, it accelerated growth and increased activity of immune cells, such as *lymphocytes, natural killers and macrophages,* and increased production of gamma-interferon, a protein with anti-viral and anti-cancer properties. The benefits of Siberian Ginseng to the immune system appear to be two-fold. Firstly, it reduces the intensity of stress response and thus protects the immune system from the ravages of stress, and secondly, it directly stimulates the activity of immune cells.

Usage: Siberian Ginseng is non-toxic and devoid of side effects in a wide range of doses. The typical dosage recommended for disease prevention and anti-aging is 2 ml of extract (the equivalent weight of dry extract is 150 mg) twice a day for a month. Such monthly cycle can be repeated 2-4 times a year. During periods of severe physical or mental stress the same dose can be taken 3-4 times a day for up to two weeks. Occasionally dried herb is used, although it is less well absorbed than the extract. The doses for dried herb usually range from 0.5 to 1.5 g 3 times a day.

CHAPTER 29

TURNING ON AFTER TURNING FIFTY

As we age, our systems inevitably enter a state of decline. However, a decline in sexuality is not an inevitable consequence of aging and fortunately it is quite preventable. Furthermore, most of the things we discuss here involving life extension contribute to preserving a healthy sexual function well into old age.

For some people, general health and youth preservation measures may still not be enough to retain sexual function. However, there are a wide range of steps you can take - from special nutrients to drugs, to injections, to penile implants - all geared towards enhancing sexual performance and desire. With existing treatments, there are certain trade-offs. Each has certain benefits as well as risks. What's more, no single method works for everyone. Nonetheless, most people should be able to find some treatment that meets their goals.

ENHANCING SEXUAL PERFORMANCE

VASODILATORS

Until recently, most treatments for erectile dysfunction were based upon the use of various vasodilators, drugs that dilate blood vessels. The activity of vasodilators dilates arteries in the penis in order to increase blood flow, and thereby causing an erection. Vasodilators widely used for impotence treatment include papaverine, phentolamine, nitroglycerine, alprostadil and others. The problem with these drugs is that they are highly effective only when directly injected into the penis. Having an injection before intercourse can seriously dampen ones' spirit, not to mention destroying the spontaneity of the moment. Also, these injections can produce both long and short-term side effects such as priapism (a persistent erection that can damage penile arteries), formation of scar tissue in the penis, headaches, hypertension and others. In light of all this, most men with erectile dysfunction tend to avoid injections, even at the expense of remaining impotent.

As an alternative to injections, some companies have developed another way of delivering vasodilators through a small catheter into the urethra. The results were mixed. The use of the drugs became a little less complicated, but the treatment also became less effective. Oral vasodilators tend to be even less effective because the dosages that are high enough to produce a significant increase in blood flow to the penis tend to cause a dramatic drop in blood pressure with severe consequences.

Topical vasodilators are only minimally effective simply because too little of the drug is absorbed through the skin.

VIAGRA

The introduction of Viagra has created worldwide mass hysteria. The rush to get it and unearth new enjoyment of life's pleasures defies anything drug manufacturers have seen before.

In fact, never in the history of prescriptive drugs has there ever been a phenomenon like it. Viagra (sildenafil) is the most promising of the recently introduced drugs for impotence and erectile dysfunction. The demand has become so great that you can now purchase it on the black market or over the Internet.

The overwhelming enthusiasm for Viagra is not without merit. Viagra was shown to improve erectile function in about 60% to 80% of men with non-organic impotence (depending on the dose in the range from 25-100 mg). Some men with mild or moderate organic impotence may also respond. In addition, Viagra appears to enhance performance in men with normal erections.

Viagra works by enhancing the effects of nitric oxide on penile arteries. The mechanism of an erection involves the release of nitric oxide in the body of the penis during sexual stimulation. Nitric oxide activates an enzyme that manufactures cyclic guanosine monophosphate (cGMP, a signaling molecule) which in turn, causes the smooth muscle in penile arteries to relax, allowing the blood to flow in the penis and cause erection. cGMP is a short-lived molecule and is quickly broken down by the enzyme phosphodiesterase type 5 (PDE 5). Viagra works by inhibiting PDE 5 which leads to elevated levels of cGMP and results in longer, firmer erections. Thus, Viagra does not cause an erection, but rather enhances an erection in response to sexual stimulation. At recommended doses, Viagra has no effect in the absence of sexual stimulation.

<u>Side Effects:</u> Viagra tends to have fewer side effects than other oral vasodilators used to treat erectile dysfunction. Side effects that were seen in clinical studies include headaches, flushing, dyspepsia (indigestion), nasal congestion and abnormal vision. Side effects increased significantly at doses higher than 100 mg.

<u>Usage:</u> Only a doctor familiar with the person's medical history should prescribe Viagra. The initial dose is usually 50 mg taken one-half to one hour before intercourse. Meals delay its onset by slowing down Viagra's absorption. Dosage may be increased to 100 mg if recommended by physician. Doses higher than 100 mg tend to produce only minimal further improvement, but cause a dramatic increase in side effects. Viagra should not be taken together with vasodilators, particularly nitrates (such as nitroglycerin) as this may cause a potentially dangerous drop in blood pressure. Dosage should be decreased in a person over sixty-five, has liver or renal impairment, or taken in combination with Tagamet (cimetidine) or erythromycin.

As of now, no studies have been done on combining Viagra with other treatments for erectile dysfunction.

ARGININE

Arginine is an essential amino acid (an indispensable building block for protein in the body) that has many effects on the body. It stimulates the release of growth hormone, enhances some aspects of the immune function and serves as a precursor in the synthesis of nitric oxide. The latter effect is responsible for the role of arginine in the mechanism of an erection because nitric oxide is a key mediator of erection needed for proper dilation of penile arteries. Studies indicate that arginine can produce a significant improvement in erectile function. In fact, arginine works along the same pathway that Viagra does. As noted in the preceding section, Viagra enhances erections by inhibiting the enzyme that destroys cGMP, a molecule that signals penile arteries to dilate. Like Viagra, arginine also increases the levels of erection-producing cGMP in the penis. It does so by increasing the production of nitric oxide that activates the enzyme producing cGMP.

Metaphorically speaking, Viagra and arginine work by filling the same bathtub. Arginine does it by opening the faucet and Viagra by blocking the drain. This relationship between the mechanisms of action of Viagra and arginine suggests that these two agents are likely to be effective in the same types of cases of erectile dysfunction. Hence for many individuals who respond to Viagra, arginine may be a safer and more affordable alternative. Theoretically, arginine might allow you to reduce the dose of Viagra without compromising its effectiveness. Presently, the combination of arginine and Viagra have not been clinically studied and should not be tried without close supervision by a physician.

Usage: When used to enhance sexual performance, arginine is usually taken about forty minutes to one hour before sexual activity. It appears that daily use of arginine, whether you engage in sex or not, enhances its overall effectiveness. The usual dose range is 1.5-5 gm. Nausea, diarrhea and stomach upset may occur at higher doses. People with serious herpes infection should not take arginine because it may stimulate the replication of the virus.

Choline and vitamin B5

An erection is a physiological event that involves not only the penis but also the brain. It all starts with sexual stimulation which is transmitted to the brain via sensory nerves. These signals are processed by the brain which sends another signal down the spinal cord to the nerves serving the penis and triggers an erection. The neurotransmitter involved in the nerve signals initiating an erection is acetylcholine. There is some evidence that increasing the production of acetylcholine in the body may potentate the nerve signals that initiate erection. Two nutrients are particularly important in this regard: choline and vitamin B5 (pantothenic acid).

Choline is a precursor of acetylcholine and the vitamin B5 is a co-enzyme required for the synthesis of acetylcholine from choline. Using these two nutrients to increase the production of acetylcholine may prolong and strengthen erections in healthy men. There is no evidence, however, that choline and vitamin B5 are useful in treating erectile dysfunction. Another noteworthy aspect of choline and B5 in regard to sexual activity is that they also increase physical endurance since acetylcholine is a key neurotransmitter. Greater endurance may also enhance sexual performance.

Usage: For enhancing sexual activity, the dosage range for choline is 1-3 gms and for vitamin B5, 0.3-1 gm (one third of that for choline). It is recommended to start at a lower end of the dosage range and gradually move up if necessary. To maximize the effects, choline and B5 should be taken about one-half hour before sexual activity. Some users report that choline and B5 appear to potentate the erection-simulating effects of arginine. Main side effects of high doses of choline and B5 are muscle tension, intestinal cramps and diarrhea which result from the action of acetylcholine in skeletal and intestinal muscles. If these effects occur, stop taking these supplements. You may try to resume after a few days at a low dose and slowly build it up.

Preventing and treating BPH

Aside from atherosclerosis, BPH (benign prostatic hypertrophy) is the main cause of sexual dysfunction in older men. Over half of all men between forty and sixty have enlarged prostate glands, a.k.a. BPH . The numbers grow even higher at more advanced ages. The main symptoms of BPH are difficulty urinating, frequent urination, nighttime awakenings to empty the bladder and, in advanced cases, complete obstruction of outflow.

Those suffering from BPH also have an increased risk of developing erectile dysfunction because an enlarged prostate may squeeze penile arteries and nerves, which interfere with the mechanism of erection. Also, surgical treatment of BPH may damage the nerve supply to the penis, resulting in impotence.

BPH is a typical age-related disease. Its incidence dramatically increases with age and is caused in part by age-related hormonal changes in the body. Particularly important are increased levels of two hormones: dihydrotestosterone and prolactin. Dihydrotestosterone (DHT) is a testosterone derivative that stimulates the growth of the prostate. Testosterone is converted to DHT by the enzyme 5-alpha reductase found in the prostate, skin and other tissues. Prolactin, a hormone produced by the pituitary gland, can intensify the rate at which the prostate takes up testosterone from the bloodstream. This indirectly contributes to BPH.

Various types of surgery are considered the main treatment in advanced cases of BPH, all of which involve a hospital stay and a risk of impotence or incontinence. A recently introduced microwave therapy holds some promise in making BPH treatment less painful and risky. It heats the prostate by using directed microwaves, to a temperature of about 40°. For unclear reasons, this results in the shrinkage of the prostate and alleviation of the symptoms. Not all patients respond and long-term results are still unclear.

The good news is that it is often possible to prevent BPH or even partially reverse mild or moderate symptoms using herbal and nutrient supplements or drugs. Interestingly, the former appears to not only be safer but more effective.

PROSCAR

Proscar' (finasteride) is the only drug currently available on the US market that has shown some effect in reducing the size of the prostate. It works by reducing the levels of DHT. Usually, Proscar must be taken for 6 months to one year to see results. In those who respond to treatment, Proscar may produce a reduction in prostate size by up to about one quarter. Proscar is a 5-mg tablet of finasteride taken once a day. Up to 5% of the patients may develop reversible impotence or decline in sexual desire.

SAW PALMETTO

Saw Palmetto (*Serenoa repens*) is a scrubby palm tree whose berries have a long history of use in folk medicine as a prostate remedy and sexual rejuvenator. In recent years, several studies have demonstrated the effectiveness of liposteroic extracts (i.e. extracts containing fats and sterols) from Saw Palmetto in reducing signs and symptoms of BPH. In fact, Saw Palmetto extract appears to be at least as effective as Proscar in reducing the size of the prostate and improving urine flow but these effects are often seen as early as 1-3 months into treatment (as opposed to up to a year with Proscar). The action of Saw Palmetto on the body is complex and appears to involve the inhibition of binding of DHT to its receptors in the prostate.

Usage: Recommended dosage for liposteroic extract of Saw Palmetto (containing at least 80% of fatty acids and sterols) is 160 mg twice a day. Consumption of dried berries or alcohol extracts is not recommended because one would have to consume very large amounts to achieve a similar effect.

Flower pollen

Flower pollen has not been studied specifically to treat BPH. However, several studies showed its effectiveness in treating the symptoms of chronic prostatitis. Recent research indicates that prostatitis often accompanies BPH and may not only account for some BPH symptoms but also contributes to its development. If pain and tenderness in the groin area are among the symptoms, some degree of prostatitis is likely.

Usage: Flower pollen extract should be used because intact pollen is only partially digested, which results in poor absorption of active ingredients. The dosage varies with the type of pollen and extract manufacturer.

Zinc

Zinc has an important role in the metabolism of the hormones that promote BPH, and is therefore critical in both prevention and successful treatment. In particular, zinc reduces negative effects of DHT on the prostate. Even mild zinc deficiency can contribute to BPH. Furthermore, zinc supplements may reduce BPH symptoms as well as prostate size in some patients. Most forms of supplemental zinc are poorly absorbed. One of the exceptions is zinc picolinate.

Usage: At high doses, zinc can be toxic. Recommended doses must not be exceeded. For BPH, most experts recommend taking 60 mg of zinc picolinate for 3 months. The dose can be reduced to 30 mg a day for another 3 months. Zinc supplements may interfere with copper absorption causing copper deficiency. Zinc supplements should be taken with copper supplements at ratio 15:1 (for each 15 mg of elemental zinc one should take 1mg of elemental copper). To avoid high doses when taking zinc-copper supplement make sure that your other vitamin and mineral supplements do not contain substantial amounts of these minerals.

RESTORING AND ENHANCING SEXUAL DRIVE AND ENJOYMENT

Aging may lead to a slackening of sexual drive (libido) and enjoyment without which sex is a chore rather than a pleasure. It is primarily caused by changes in the central nervous system as well as hormonal shifts. In many cases, these changes can be counteracted and sex drive restored to a more youthful state. Particularly important in maintaining a healthy sex drive is the condition of the central aging clock. Many nutrients and drugs that help "rewind" the central aging clock, particularly those that raise dopamine levels in the hypothalamus, appear to enhance sex drive.

The intensity of sensations during sex is partly dependent on the brain and partly on local environment around nerve endings in the genital and erogenous zones. Viagra and arginine are not just pro-erection agents. They enhance sexual enjoyment in both men and women by increasing blood flow to genital areas.

NIACIN

Niacin (nicotinic acid), a vitamin, when taken in doses over 100 mg produces an effect resembling "sex flush." It does so by stimulating histamine release (which in turn causes dilation of blood vessels in the skin) seen as a flush. Histamine release often occurs spontaneously during sexual excitation producing a natural sexual flush. Niacin, however, can substantially intensify the effect and more importantly, can dramatically increase sensation all over the body as well as in the genital area. Erogenous stimulation and orgasm may become much more intense. Niacin may even help some people who have trouble achieving orgasm because histamine has a role in experiencing orgasm.
Usage: To enhance sexual enjoyment, niacin is best taken on an empty stomach. Niacin flush usually occurs fifteen to thirty minutes after ingestion and lasts for ten to twenty minutes. For best results, you may want to be at the peak of the flush at the time of orgasm. For

people who do not use niacin on a daily basis, doses as small as 100 mg or even less may produce this flush. However, tolerance develops quickly with regular use. Niacin is acidic and may cause acid indigestion. To prevent this, take it with an antacid or wash it down with a solution of baking soda in water. High doses of niacin (over 800 mg a day or over 200 as a single dose) can cause liver problems and should not be taken without a doctors supervision. Diabetics should not take niacin as it may raise blood sugar. In some people, niacin may cause a sudden drop in blood pressure, especially in those taking high blood pressure medications.

YOHIMBE AND YOHIMBINE

Yohimbe (*Coryanthe yohimbe*) is a plant native to West Africa. Some tribes in the region use a brew from the bark of yohimbe to enhance male virility and sexual prowess. Western explorers reported that local tribes used the bark of yohimbe in tribal sex ceremonies that involved intense sexual activity and lasted for as long as 2 weeks. The observers' opinion was that this brew made such extraordinary sexual activity possible.

In recent decades, there has been a considerable amount of research on yohimbe. Most studies were made not with yohimbe bark itself, but with the purified active ingredient yohimbine. Studies investigating the use of yohimbine in treating impotence produced mixed findings. Some studies in men with organic impotence (i.e. mainly those with penile blood vessel obstruction or nerve damage) concluded that yohimbine was no better than a placebo. Other studies reported certain limited benefits. Studies involving men with non-organic impotence had a somewhat better response. An overall picture appears to be that yohimbine is more effective in cases of mild, short-term non-organic impotence. The effects of yohimbine appear to be greatest in men with healthy or slightly declining sexual function in whom it increases sex drive. It makes erections easier to obtain and maintain and produces a more powerful orgasm. Thus yohimbine is more an aphrodisiac than a drug for organic impotence. In fact, yohimbine was the first drug ever to be described in *Physician's Desk Reference* (a pharmacology bible for US physicians) as an agent that "may have activity as an aphrodisiac."

<u>Side effects:</u> A frequent side effect of yohimbine and yohimbe is anxiety, most common at very high doses, but may also occur at lower doses. Other reported side effects include: high blood pressure, tremor, nausea vomiting, rapid heart rate, excessive salivation and sweating, overstimulation, irritability, lack of coordination, headaches and flushing. Normal doses, however, usually produce little or no side effects in healthy people. Yohimbine or yohimbe should not be used by geriatric patients, pregnant women, children, psychiatric patients, and people with kidney problems or people with history of peptic ulcer. Yohimbine or yohimbe should not be used in combination with antidepressants or other mood-altering drugs and should only be used with extreme caution in people treated for or with a history of high blood pressure.

<u>Usage:</u> Yohimbine is considered a drug and must be prescribed by a physician. Many people use the alternative, yohimbe bark sold over-the-counter in health food stores. Researchers Morgenthaler and Joy in their 1995 book "Better Sex Through Chemistry" state that there is evidence that most quality brands of yohimbe contain at least as much yohimbine per capsule as prescription yohimbine tablets. Yohimbine tablets contain 5.4 mgs each, doses reportedly used in treatment of erectile dysfunction range from 3 - 8 tablets a day (16.2 - 43.2 mg per day). The yohimbine content in commonly sold yohimbe capsules varies widely and may be several times higher than in one yohimbine tablet. People who consider using yohimbe capsules for occasional sexual enhancement should try very low doses first (less than a capsule dosage can be obtained by opening the capsule and removing some of the powder). The dose can be gradually and cautiously adjusted until the desired effect is obtained or any side effects develop. Effects of a yohimbine dose are usually seen within an hour. Some effects of yohimbine may accumulate over several days with repeated use.

CHAPTER 30

AGELESS BEAUTY.

Like it or not, our physical appearance has tremendous impact on our lives. We live in a society in which physical beauty is often considered more important than intelligence. This is in good part due to our media-driven culture fueled by Hollywood as well as television. However, our evolutionary past also plays some role. In the wild, animals strive to find a mate with an optimal genetic makeup to give their offspring the best possible chance of survival. The animal, however, gives no thought to Darwinian evolution and genetics. Its partner selection mechanisms are genetically programmed. The visual image of a prospective mate, along with its smell and behavior are the inputs the brain subconsciously processes to determine a genetically suitable mate. Physical beauty indicates the absence of genetic flaws and diseases and a youthful appearance shows that the prospective mate is able to reproduce.

Whatever the reasons, social, biological or just pure peer pressure, most of us strive to look young and appealing. It raises our self-esteem, lifts our spirits, improves our chances with the opposite sex and according to some studies, it makes others treat us better.

Beauty is only skin deep, depending upon the condition of the skin, that is. Skin is the single largest organ in the human body and suffers the same age-related damage from free radicals, cross-linking and hormonal shifts as the rest of the body. In addition, skin is directly exposed to the environment and damaged by ultraviolet radiation and pollutants.

General measures in retarding the aging process described in other chapters will also help slow down skin aging and may even improve its appearance. Supplemental antioxidants like vitamins C and E, selenium, cysteine, flavonoids (found in plant sources, e.g., grape seeds), and polyphenols (found in green tea) may shift the damage-repair equilibrium towards skin rejuvenation. People starting on reasonably high doses of antioxidants often notice improved skin elasticity and texture within a few weeks.

UV-light is one of the main culprits in premature aging of the skin. UV rays generate free radicals and induces cross-linking (abnormal bridges between molecules), causing wrinkles, loss of smoothness and elasticity. The surest way to protect your skin is by avoiding exposure to the sun. An alternative is using sunscreen but most sunscreens do relatively little to prevent skin from aging. There are two types of ultraviolet light, UVA and UVB. Sunburn is caused mainly by UVB. Skin aging, wrinkles and skin cancer are caused mainly by UVA. Light with different frequencies tends to attack different components within the skin. Most sunscreen, especially those with SPF higher than 15, are very good at protecting your skin from the harmful effects of UVB, but offer little or no protection against UVA so they do not help prevent wrinkles or reduce the risk of skin cancer. When shopping for a sunscreen make sure that it has an SPF of 15 or higher, and that it offers protection against both UVA and UVB. The best sunscreen includes an effective UVA blocker such as avobenzone, titanium dioxide, and zinc oxide.

When venturing outdoors, don't assume that wearing a hat or staying in the shade can protect you from UV light. Reflected light may retain over a third of its UV rays. When outside always wear a UVA & UVB-blocking sunscreen.

You may have heard that glass blocks UV rays. It may block UVB rays quite well, but doesn't block UVA rays. As odd as it sounds, in a room bright with natural light you would be wise to wear sunscreen to ensure maximum UV protection.

Some people choose to stay out of the sun. This is clearly a solution for minimizing UV damage, but it does have a significant downside (in addition to reducing your enjoyment of life). In some people, lack of exposure to daylight may disturb normal sleep patterns, leading to insomnia and depression. (This has to do with the effect of light on the production of serotonin and melatonin.) Sunlight is also needed by the body for vitamin D, a deficiency which leads to bone loss and poor immunity. If you have no exposure to the sun, make sure that you get 100% RDA for vitamin D in your vitamin supplement in vitamin D fortified milk.

UV rays are not the only factors that accelerate the skin aging. Heavy drinking and smoking don't usually go hand in hand with young looking skin. Acetaldehyde, a product of alcohol metabolism, and tobacco smoke substances are potent cross-linkers that prematurely age the skin along with other organs. Diabetes or poor glucose tolerance also contribute to skin aging because high glucose levels accelerate both cross-linking and the formation of free radicals. Steps to improve your carbohydrate tolerance, such as attaining optimal weight, a high fiber diet, exercise, and supplemental chromium reduces the risk of degenerative-diseases and may also help delay skin wrinkling. In postmenopausal women, estrogen replacement often remarkably improves skin texture and elasticity. Restoring the youthful levels of growth hormone was reported to modestly increase skin thickness in both sexes.

All of the above, except for avoiding or blocking UV-rays, are a part of the basic anti-aging strategy for the body as a whole. But the skin is special, not only for our self-image, but because of its accessibility. Is there anything we can do specifically for our skin? Are there any valid anti-aging cosmetic products or procedures available today? Is there something that can actually reverse visible signs of aging - soften wrinkles, reduce facial sag, eliminate age spots and blemishes? The number of clinical studies on skin rejuvenation is surprisingly small. As of today, several topical treatments such as retinoids, alpha-hydroxy acids and estrogens have consistently shown to reverse skin aging to some degree. We will not be discussing invasive methods like surgery, laser resurfacing, botulinum toxin injections, or deep chemical peels. These methods are excluded from the content of this book because their aim is reconstruction rather than rejuvenation. Albeit expensive and often painful, these methods may be valuable for image preservation. However, we advise that both the risks and benefits of invasive or aggressive skin treatments be carefully explored before taking any steps.

ALPHA HYDROXY ACIDS

Alpha-hydroxy acids (AHA) are a group of structurally related organic acids mainly from plant sources. AHA was found to improve skin wrinkling, elasticity and texture by reversing some of the processes seen in aging skin.

As we age, the skin becomes thinner and more fragile, primarily because cell division slows down and production of collagen and elastin (key structural proteins of the skin) decline. AHA was found to combat skin aging by peeling off excess dead cells (keratinocytes) and more importantly, by stimulating the growth and thickening of the dermis and epidermis; the two main layers of the skin.

While the way it works is unclear, several studies have showed that AHA indeed had some potential to reverse the signs of aging skin.

In a 1996 study conducted by Dr. Newman and colleagues in California, 45 volunteers were treated with 50% glycolic acid. The treatment was applied to one side of the face, forearms and hands for 5 minutes once weekly for 1 month. The researchers concluded that a significant improvement was noted, including a decrease in rough texture and fine wrinkling, fewer solar keratoses and a slight lightening of solar lentigines. Histology showed thinning of stratum corneum (the outermost skin layer consisting mostly of dead cells), granular layer enhancement and epidermal thickening. The results of this study demonstrate that the application of 50% glycolic acid peels improves mild photo aging of the skin.

In another study, Dr. Ditre and colleagues from Hahnemann University School of Medicine tested a lotion containing 2% of gly colic, lactic or citric acids against a placebo lotion. The treatment was continued for 6 months. AHA treatment led to a 25% increase in skin thickness, improved quality of elastic fibers and increased density of collagen. The research concluded that AHA "produced a significant reversal of epidermal and dermal markers of photoaging."

Many AHA-based creams and lotions are available over the counter. Most of these products contain relatively low concentrations of AHA, usually 5%-15%. Massachusetts General Hospital in Boston studied the efficacy of low-strength topical AHA preparations (8% glycolic and 8% lactic acid lotions). The study was conducted on 74 women aged forty to seventy, with moderately severe photodamaged facial skin. The creams were applied twice daily for 22 weeks. The percentage of patients achieving at least 1 grade of improvement on 0-9 scale was 76% for glycolic acid, 71% for lactic acid, and 40% for placebo vehicle. The researchers concluded that low-strength AHA preparations were "modestly useful" for reversing some of the signs of skin aging.

When using commercial AHA-based skin care products, be sure the AHA content is at least 8%. Use these products consistently, at least once a day and apply to thoroughly washed skin to ensure good absorption. High strength AHA preparations may be more effective. However, because of the greater potential for skin irritation, they should only be used under the supervision of a dermatologist.

There is one caution to be made about alpha-hydroxy acid. The main benefits come from its ability to exfoliate skin. Removal of the outermost layer of skin stimulates the cells in lower layers to grow and divide, causing the skin to thicken and in the process, diminishes visible signs of aging. The more you exfoliate the more cell divisions will occur in the lower skin layers. The problem is that normal human cells cannot divide indefinitely. Fibroblasts (a key type of cells in the skin) would divide about 50 times and then enter a stage of senescence as they approach the Hayflick limit. This is a state in which the cell is sluggish, inefficient, unresponsive to various signals from the body and unable to divide. Skin with many such cells is usually fragile, blotchy and easily wrinkled. Exfoliation with AHA or other methods remains a valuable cosmetic tool but overuse it and your skin may "hit the Hayflick limit" earlier than it should.

Tretinoin

Retin A (Tretinoin) is a form of retinoic acid that is an active derivative of vitamin A. Retinoic acid produces multiple effects in various organs, including the skin. In particular, it increases the responsiveness of skin cells to epidermal growth factor (EGF), the natural hormone that stimulates skin growth.

The anti-aging effect of topical Retin A on the skin has been documented in many well-designed studies. Retin A was found to reduce fine wrinkles and skin roughness, increase epidermal thickness and stimulate deposition of collagen. In one study 0.05% Retin A cream was found superior to 6% glycolic acid in improving skin elasticity. Typical strength of topical Retin A creams is 0.025-0.1%. With Retin A, like many things, more isn't always better. One study found that 0.025% Retin A may be as effective as 0.05%-0.1%, but with lower incidence of skin irritation. For people with sensitive skin, 0.25% may be the optimal strength. According to the studies, improvement by Retin A may continue for up to a year of continued use.

Technically, retinoic acid may be considered a nutrient because it is a natural metabolite of vitamin A. It is also present in trace amounts in some foods of animal origin. However, significant doses of retinoic acid taken orally may cause severe side effects resembling vitamin A overdose. Retinoic acid creams, such as topical Retin A, do not have any significant systemic action. Their main side effect is skin irritation. At present, topical Retin A is sold by prescription.

ESTROGENS

It has been noted that after menopause women begin to age more rapidly. Wrinkles spread faster while skin quickly loses elasticity and smoothness. To a large degree this seems to result from the decline of estrogen levels during menopause. Of all the hormones that decline with age, estrogens have the most dramatic effect on the skin. Estrogens are known to protect women from heart disease and now it seems that they also slow down skin aging. Several studies indicate that postmenopausal women on estrogen replacement therapy develop fewer wrinkles and have better skin texture and elasticity than those not on estrogens.

While estrogen replacement is a complex decision requiring the analysis of one's medical history. Dr. Schmidt and colleagues in Vienna studied the effects of topical estrogen treatment with 0.01% estradiol or 0.3% estriol in 59 postmenopausal women. After six months of treatment, a marked improvement in skin elasticity and firmness was noted; wrinkle depth and pore size decreased by over 60% in both groups, Skin moisture and collagen synthesis increased significantly. No systemic effects caused by estrogens were observed.

Theoretically, estrogen creams also alleviate the signs of aging in premenopausal women and in men, although there have been no clinical studies to confirm this. Various prescriptions and over-the-counter estrogen based creams are commercially available.

TOPICAL ANTIOXIDANTS

Skin is highly susceptible to free radical damage through its constant exposure to the environment and high content of unsaturated fatty acids. Topical antioxidants provide some protection from environmental damage and may be somewhat effective in slowing down skin aging. One of the commonly used formulas is a combination of vitamins C and E, a water and fat-soluble antioxidant. Vitamin C is also involved in the synthesis of collagen, a major structural protein in the skin, which may help improve skin texture. Vitamin A, another common ingredient of cosmetic products is also modestly useful. It serves as an antioxidant and a precursor for the synthesis of retinoic acid (see above). It is important to note that commercial antioxidant-containing ointments have a limited shelf life. Antioxidants are easily inactivated by oxygen from air, especially at warm temperatures and when exposed to light. When purchasing antioxidant creams, be sure to check the expiration date. Containers should be kept in a dark, cool place, tightly sealed.

Na-PCA

Skin aging is also associated with the gradual loss of moisture. Dry skin wrinkles more easily, is less elastic, has weaker repair mechanisms and looks older as well. The skin's principal natural moisturizer is sodium 2-pyrrolidone-5-carboxylate or Na-PCA. The skin levels of Na-PCA in older people are about one-half of those in young people. Restoring Na-PCA levels can markedly improve the appearance of dry skin. Some commercial skin creams and moisturizers, usually the more expensive ones include Na-PCA. Check labels for the list of ingredients.

CHAPTER 31

COPING WITH STRESS IN THE POST 9/11 WORLD

On September 11, 2001, life as we know it in America changed forever. The terrorist attack launched against the World Trade Center robbed us of the peace and tranquility we once took for granted. In its wake, there are now growing fears over bio-terrorism, a faltering economy, and the constant threat of a nation besieged by terrorism.

We grieve for the many thousands of people who lost their lives and the families they left behind. Unfortunately, they were not the only victims. In a recent survey, it was reported that 7% of the population is now suffering from some form of post traumatic stress disorder. PTSD first gained recognition in veterans returning from the Vietnam War. In a sense, it is the human body reacting to an overwhelming event or some extremely stressful situation. PTSD is often characterized by a wide range of nonspecific symptoms such as listlessness, sleep deprivation, loss of appetite, avoidance of large crowds, and a hypersensitivity to loud noises. It is unusual in that it is difficult to diagnose and may not show itself immediately.

It is no mere coincidence that many of these symptoms are identical to those found in depression. Both PTSD and depression are associated with abnormalities in the stress response mechanism. Many people experienced some or all of these symptoms during the period immediately following 9/11, but as they returned to their normal daily routines, the symptoms gradually dissipated. However, in some cases these symptoms have lingered on or even escalated over time.

If you or someone you know is suffering from some or all of these symptoms, it would be wise to seek professional help or counseling.

Similar to depression, PTSD intensifies several mechanisms of aging. In both cases, the body appears to be thrown into a state resembling chronic stress. The sympathetic nervous system releases anxiety hormones (epinephrine and norepinephrine) which can cause rapid heartbeat, palpitations, muscular tension and nausea.

The biological relationship between depression, stress and aging is discussed in detail in previous chapters. Here we would like to focus on some practical things you can do to help mitigate and potentially overcome the everyday stresses in this extraordinarily stressful world. Keep in mind, regardless of the severity of its symptoms, PTSD requires qualified professional help.

Exercise

Moderate exercise 3 - 5 times a week is not only beneficial to the body, but also the spirit. In addition to releasing tension, activities like jogging, swimming, and weight training release endorphins, promote a healthy immune system and improve self-esteem. Even a brisk walk can prove beneficial in terms of reducing stress, improving heart function and overall health. Physical activity in general, whether exercise or work related is a good way to reduce pent up tension, keep the immune system in good shape, and provide a better sense of well-being.

Meditation and Bio Feedback

Another method of reducing tension and stress is through meditation. We have nothing against burning incense or sitting in a lotus position. However, the kind of meditation we are referring to requires no knowledge of yoga - just a nice comfortable chair in a relatively quiet place.

Start by closing your eyes and building a picture in your mind of some idyllic spot - a warm sandy beach, a picturesque snow-covered mountain or even a quiet spot by a lake. As this picture solidifies, take deep breaths, hold them for a moment, and then exhale slowly. This tends to reduce blood pressure and heart rate and thus reduces your body's secretion of stress hormone (cortisol). In other words, it helps you achieve a better sense of equilibrium in body and mind.

Biofeedback, a more elaborate cousin of meditation, is a computer aided technique that enables you to help control certain involuntary body functions such as blood pressure, heart rate and skin temperature. This method employs a computerized device that helps you to "visualize" these functions. In the process, you "learn" to bring these involuntary functions into a more "normal" range.

ADAPTOGENS

As discussed in Chapter 28, adaptogens are among the most effective weapons in combating stress. They optimize resistance to a wide variety of stress factors and enhance the body's ability to recover from stress unscathed.

It is important to note that adaptogens, among other things, modify the body's stress response, enabling faster recovery. In particular, some adaptogens, such as Siberian Ginseng, reduce the intensity of the alarm phase of the stress response, thus reducing stress related damage. Also, many adpatogens (ginseng, Siberian Ginseng, and others) improve metabolism, even in a non-stressful environment. This enhances both physical and mental endurance. In fact, the metabolic effects of ginseng are in some ways similar to the effects of physical exercise. In other words, ginseng may be the closest you can come to working out without giving up your status as a "couch potato." Unfortunately, you cannot obtain all the healthy benefits of exercise by just taking ginseng supplements.

Other lesser know adaptogens also include Indian Ginseng, holy basil, gold root, scizandra and leuzea. But before you embark on a course of taking adaptogens, please refer to Chapter 28.

VITAMINS AND MINERALS

During periods of prolonged stress you may have elevated levels of stress hormones in your blood stream. Stress hormones accelerate the depletion of the body's stores of several vitamins and minerals, particularly potassium, pantothenic acid, and vitamins C and B6. During stressful times it is especially important to maintain a diet high in these nutrients.

Melatonin may prove helpful in the treatment of sleep disorders, hypertension, and a decreased immunity - all of which can be induced or exacerbated by stress or emotional trauma.

All said, there is literally nothing anyone can do to change the events that took place on 9/11. It is something we will live with for the rest of our lives. However, post-traumatic stress disorder doesn't have to be a part of it.

REFERENCES

Note from the authors: While writing this book, we went through literally hundreds of research articles and other publications. Since our work is meant for a general audience rather than serious students, you will find only a partial list of references that include what we believe to be the most relevant material. We apologize for any omissions.

Ames, B.N., Shigenaga, M.K., Hagen, T.M. *Oxidants, antioxidants, and the degenerative-diseases of aging*. Proc Natl Acad Sci USA 90:7915-7922,1993.

Bachmann, G.A. *Influence of menopause on sexuality*. Int J Fertil Menopausal Stud, 40,Suppl 1:16-22,1995.

Baltrusch, H.J., Stangel, W., Titze, I. *Stress, cancer and immunity. New developments in biopsychosocial and psychoneuroimmunologic research*. Acta Neurol (Napoli), Aug,13:4, 315-27,1991.

Bjorntorp, P. *Neuroendocrine ageing*.(Review). Journal of Internal Medicine, 238(5):401-4, 1995.

Bouillanne, O., Rainfray, M., Tissandier, O. et al. *Growth hormone therapy in elderly people: an age-delaying drug?* Fundam Clin Pharmacol 10:5, 416-30,1996.

Brindley, D.N., Rolland, Y. *Possible connections between stress, diabetes, obesity, hypertension and altered lipoprotein metabolism that may result in atherosclerosis*.Clin Sci 77:5, 453-61, 1989.

Bryla, C.M. *The relationship between stress and the development of breast cancer: a literature review*. Oncol Nurs Forum, Apr, 23:3, 441-8, 1996.

Bu-Abbas, A., Clifford, M.N., Walker, R. et al. *Marked antimutagenic potential of aqueous green tea extract: mechanism of action*. Mutagenesis, Jul, 9:4, 325-31,1994.

Burnett, A.L., Lowenstein, C.J., Bredt, D.S., et al. *Nitric Oxide, a physiologic mediator of penial erection*. Science 257:401-4, 1992.

Casper, R.C. *Nutrition and its relationship to aging*. Exp Gerontol, May-Aug, 30:3-4, 299-314,1995.

Chrousos, G., Gold, Ph. W. *The concepts of stress and stress system disorders. Overview of physical and behavioral homeostasis*. JAMA, 267:1244-1252, 1992.

Conti, A., Maestroni, G.I. *The clinical neuroimmunotherapeutic role of melatonin in oncology*. J Pineal Res, Oct, 19:3, 103-10, 1995.

Comfort, A., Dial, L.K. Sexuality and aging. An overview. Clin Geriatr Med Feb, 7:1, 1-7,1991.

Counter, C.M. *The roles of telomeres and telomerase in cell life span*. Mutat Res, Oct, 366:1, 45-63, 1996.

Curtsinger, J.W., Fukui, H.H., Khazaeli, A.A. et al. *Genetic variation and aging*. Annu Rev Genet 29:553-75, 1995.

Dilman, V.M. Development, Aging, and Disease. *A new Rationale for an Intervention Strategy*. Harwood Academic Publishers, 1994.

Dinan, T.G. *Noradrenergic and serotonergic abnormalities in depression: stress-induced dysfunction?* J Clin Psychiatry, 57 Suppl 4:14-8,1996.

Van Eekelen, J.A., Rots, N.Y., Sutanto, W. et al. *The effect of aging on stress responsiveness and central corticosteroid receptors in the brown Norway rat*. Neurobiol Aging, Jan-Feb, 13:1, 159-70,1992.

Eysenck, H.J. *Personality, stress and cancer: prediction and prophylaxis*. Br J Med Psychol Mar, 61 (Pt.1):57-75, 1988.

Fawcett, T.W., Sylvester, S.L., Sarge, K.D. et al. *Effects of neurohormonal stress and aging on the activation of mammalian heat shock factor 1*. J Biol Chem 269:51, 32272-8, 1994.

Fontenot, M.B., Kaplan, J.R., Manuck, S.B. et al. *Long-term effects of cronic social stress on serotonergic indices in the prefrontal cortex of adult male cynomolgus macaques*. Brain Res 705:1-2,105-8,1995.

Fowler, C.J., Wiberg, A., Oreland, L. et al. *The effect of age and molecular properties of human brain monoamine oxidase*. J Neurol Transm 49:1-2, 1-20, 1980.

Frolkis, V.V. *Stress-age syndrome*. Mech Ageing Dev Jun ,69:1-2, 93-107, 1993.

Frolkis, V.V. *Syndromes of aging.(Review)*. Gerontology, 38(1-2):80-6,1992.

Garcia-Patterson, A., Puig-Domingo, M., Webb, S.M. *Thirty years of human pineal research:do we know its clinical relevance?* J Pineal Res , Jan, 20:1, 1-6, 1996.

Gilad, G.M., Gilad, V.H. *Strain, stress, neurodegeneration and longevity*. Mech Ageing Dev, Mar 1,78:2,75-83, 1995.

Graeff, F.G., Guimares, F.S., De Andrade, T.G. et al. *Role of 5-HT in stress, anxiety, and depression*. Pharmacol. Biochem Behav, May, 54:1, 129-41, 1996.

Harman, D. *Aging and disease: extending functional lifespan*. Ann NY Acad Sci, 786:, 321-36, 1996.

Hassig, A., Wen-Xi, L., Stampfli, K. *Stress-induced suppression of the cellular immune reactions: on the neuroendocrine control of the immune system*. Med Hypothesis, Jun, 46:6, 551-5, 1996.

Herman, J.P., Prewitt, C.M., Collinan, W.E. *Neuronal circuit regulation of hypothalamopituitary-adrenocortical stress axis*. Crit Rev Neurobiol 10:3-4, 371-94, 1996.

Heydari, A.R., Takahashi, R., Gutsmann, A. et al. *Hsp 70 and aging*. Experientia Nov 30, 50:11-12,1092-8,1994.

Huether, G. *Melatonin as an antiaging drug: between facts and fantasy*. Gerontology, 42:2, 87-96,1996.

Iannidou-Mouzaka, L., Mantonakis, J., Toufexi, H. et al. *Is prolonged psychological stress an ethiological factor in breast cancer?* J Gynecol Obstet Biol Reprod (Paris), 15:8, 1049-53,1986.

Jacobson, L., Sapolsky, R. *The role of hyppocampus in feedback regulation of the hypothalamic-pituitary-adrenocortical axis*. Endocr Rev, May, 12:2, 118-34,1991.

Jenkins, R.R. *Exercise, oxidative stress, and antioxidants: a review*. International Journal of Sport Nutrition 3(4):356-75, Dec 1993.

Jensen, G.D., Polloi, A.H. *The very old of Palau: health and mental state*. Age Aging, Jul ,17:4, 220-6, 1988.

Johannsson, G., MArin, P., Lonn, L. et al. *Growth hormone treatment of abdominally obese men reduces abdominal fat mass, improves glucose and lipoprotein metabolism, and reduces diastolic blood pressure.* J Clin Metab Mar, 82:3, 727-34,1997.

Johnson, M.A., Brown, M.A., Poon, L.W. et al. *Nutritional patterns of cen-*

tenarians. Int J Aging Hum Dev 34:1, 57-76, 1992.

Kauffman, S.H. *Heat shock proteins in health and disease. (Review)*. International Journal of Clinical & Laboratory Research 21(3):221-6, 1992.

Khan, R., Daya, S., Potgieter, B. *Evidence for a modulation of the stress response by the pineal gland*. Experientia Aug 15, 46:8, 860-2,1990.

Khorram, O., Vu, L., Yen ,S.S. *Activation of immune function by dehydroepiandrosterone (DHEA) in age-advanced men*. J Gerontol A Biol Sci Med Sci, Jan, 52:1, M1-7,1997.

Klatz, R. and Kahn, C. *Grow Young with HGH*. Harper Collins Publishers, 1997.

Lechin, F., Van der Dijs, B., Benaim, M. *Stress versus depression*. Prog Neuropsychopharmacol Biol Psychiatry Aug, 20:6, 899-950, 1996.

Lee, Y.K., Manalo, D., Liu. A.Y. *Heat shock response, heat shock transcription factor and cell aging*.Biol Signals, May-June, 5:3, 180-91, 1996.

Leonard, B.E., Song, C. *Stress and immune system in the ethiology of anxiety and depression*. Pharmacol Biochem Behav, May, 54:1, 299-303, 1996.

Life, Stress and Coronary Heart Disease by Ulf De Faire, Tores Theorell, Warren H.Green, Inc, St. Louis, Missouri, USA.

Lipartiti, M., Franceschini, D., Zanoni, R.et al. *Neuroprotective effects of melatonin*. Adv Exp Med Biol 398:, 315-21, 1996.

Liu, A.Y., Lee, Y.K., Manalo, D. et al. *Attenuated heat shock transcriptional response in aging: molecular mechanism and implication in the biology of aging*. EXS, 77:, 393-408,1996.

Lonn, L., Johansson, G., Sjostrom, L. et al. *Body composition and tissue distribution in growth hormone deficient adults before and after growth hormone treatment*. Obes Res, Jan, 4:1,45-54,1996.

Maestroni, G.J. *The immunoneuroendocrine role of melatonin*. J Pineal Res Jan, 14:1,1-10, 1993.

McFarland, G.A., Holliday, R. *Retardation of the senescence of cultured human diploid fibroblasts by carnosine*. Exp Cell Res, Jun, 212:2, 167-75, 1994.

Meerson, F.Z. *Adaptogenes, Stress and Prevention*. Moscow: Nauka, 1981 (in Russian).

Miquel, J., de Juan, E., Sevila,I. *Oxigen-induced mitohondrial damage and aging*. EXS, 62:,47-57,1992.

Mimura, G., Murakami, K., Gushiken, M. *Nutritional factors for longevity in Okinavapresent and future.* Nutr Health, 8:2-3, 159-63, 1992.

Mizock, B.A. *Alteration in carbohydrate metabolism during stress: a review of the literature.* American Journal of Medicine, 98(1):75-84, Jan, 1995.

Mocchegiani, E., Paolucci, P., Balsamo, A. et al. *Influence of growth hormone on thymic endocrine activity in humans.* Horm Res 33:6, 248-55, 1990.

Modern Nutrition in Health and Disease, edited by M.E.Shils, J.A.Olson, and M.Shike, 8th ed. Lea & Fabiger, 1994.

Morgenthaler, J., Joy, D. *Better Sex Through Chemistry: A guide to new prosexual drugs.* Petaluma, CA: Smart Publications, 1995.

Murray, M., and J.Pizzorno. *Encyclopedia of Natural Medicine.* Prima Publishing, 1991.

Oreland, L., Gottfries, C.G. *Brain and brain monoamine oxidase in aging and in dementia of Alzheimer's type.* Prog Neuropsychopharmacol Biol Psychiatry, 10:3-5,533-40, 1986.

Packer, L., Tritschler, H.J., Wessel, K. *Neuroprotection by the metabolic antioxidant alpha-lipoic acid.* Free Radic Biol Med 22:1-2, 359-78, 1997.

Parsons, P.A. *The limit to human longevity: an approach through a stress theory of ageing.* Mech Ageing Dev, Jun 25, 87:3, 211-8, 1996.

Pearson, D., and Show, S. *Life extension. A practical scientific approach.* Warner Books, 1983.

Perls, T.T. *The oldest old.* Scintific American 272: No.1, 70-75, 1995.

Ravaglia, G., Forti, P., Maioli, F. et al. *The relationship of dehydroepiandrosterone sulfate (DHEAS) to endocrine-metabolic parameters and functional status in the oldest-old. Results from an Italian study on healthy free-living over-ninety-year-olds.* J Clin Endocrinol Metab, Mar., 81:3, 1173-8, 1996.

Receputo, G., Rapisarda, R., Motta, L. *Centenarians: health status and life conditions.* Ann Ital Med Int, Jan-Mar, 10:1, 41-5, 1995.

Reiter, R.J., and Robinson J. *Melatonin.* Bantam Books, 1996.

Regelson, W., Kalimi M. *Dehydroepiandrosterone (DHEA) the multifunctional steroid.II. Effects on the CNS, cell proliferation, metabolic and vascular, clinical and other effects. Mechanism of action.* Ann NY Acad Sci 719, 564-575.

Rothuizen, J., Reul, J.M., Rijnberk, A. et al. *Aging and hypothalamus-pitu-*

itaryadrenocortical axis, with special reference to the dog. Acta Endocrinol (Copenh.), 125, Suppl I, 73-6, 1991.

Rudman, D., Feller, A.G., Cohn L. et al. *Effects of human growth hormone on body composition in elderly men*. Horm Res 36 Suppl 1:, 73-81, 1991.

Sahelian, R. *DHEA. A practical Guide*. Garden City Park, 1996.

Sardesai, V.M. *Role of antioxidants in health mainteance*. Nutr Clin Pract, Feb, 10:1, 19-25, 1995.

Schlesinger, M.J. *How the cell copes with stress and the function of heat shock proteins*. Pediatric Research, 36 (1Pt.1):1-6, Jul, 1994.

Serafini, M., Ghiselli, A., Ferro-Luzzi, A. *In vivo antioxidant effect of green and black tea in man*. Eur J Clin Nutr, Jan, 50:1, 28-32, 1996.

Sohal, R.S., Weindruch, R. *Oxidative stress, caloric restriction, and aging*. Science, Jul 5, 273:5271, 59-63, 1996.

Stokes, P.E. *The potential role of excessive cortisol induced by HPA hyperfunction in the pathogenesis of depression*. Eur Neuropsychopharmacol, 5 Suppl:, 77-82, 1995.

Stress and Heart Disease, ed. by E.Beamish, P.K.Singal, N.S.Dhalla, Martinus Nijhoff Publishing, Boston, 1984.

Svendsen, L., Rattan, S.I., Clark, B.F. *Testing garlic for possible anti-aging effects on long-term growth characteristics, morphology and macromolecular synthesis of human fibroblasts in culture*. J Ethnopharmacol, Jul 8, 43:2, 125-33, 1994.

Todorov, I.N. *How cells maintain stability*. Scientific American Dec, 66-75, 1990.

Todorov, I.N. *Mechanism of antistress and anabolic actions of eleutherococcus senticosus maximum extracts.In Bioactive Compounds: Biotransformation and Biological Action*, edited by I.N.Todorov, G.E.Zaikov, and A.Degterev, Nova Science Publishers, Inc., 1993.

Todorov I.N., *Mechanism of cell stability: subcellular and molecular aspects*. Nova Science Publishers, Inc, 1993.

Tsitouras,P.D., Bulat, T. *The aging male reproductive system*. Endocrinol Metab Clin North Am, Jun, 24:2, 297-315, 1995.

Ursin, H. *Stress, distress and immunity*. Annals NY Academy of Sciences, 204-211,1994.

Vijg, J., Wei, J.Y. *Understanding the biology of aging: the key to prevention and therapy.* J Am Geriatr Soc, Apr, 43:4, 426-34, 1995.

Villareal, D.T., Morley, J.E. *Trophic factors in aging. Should older people receive hormonal replacement therapy?* Drugs Aging, Jun , 4:6,492-509, 1994.

Wachs, T.D. *Relation of mild-to-moderate malnutrition to human development: correlational studies.* J Nutr, Aug, 125:8 Suppl, 2245S-2254S, 1995.

Wiley, D., Bortz, W.M.2nd. *Sexuality and aging-usual and successful.* J Gerontol A Biol Sci, May, 51:3, M142-6, 1996.

Wilson, J.D., and Foster, D.W. *Textbook of Endocrinology, 7th ed.* W.B.Saunders Company, 1985.

Wolkovitz, O.M., Reus, V.I., Roberts, E. et al. *Dehydroepiandrosterone (DHEA) treatment of depression.* Biol Psychiatry, Feb 1, 41:3, 311-8, 1997.

Yen, S.S.,Morales, A.J., Khorram, O. *Replacement of DHEA in aging men and women. Potential remedial effects.* Ann NY Acad Sci Dec 29, 774, 128-42, 1995.

Yin, D. *Biochemical basis of lipofuscin, ceroid, and age pigment-like fluorophores.* Free Radic Biol Med, 21:6, 871-88, 1996.

Yin, D. *Studies on age pigments evolving into a new theory of biological aging.* Gerontlogy 41 Suppl 2:, 159-72, 1995.

Yu, B.P. *Aging and oxidative stress: modulation by dietary restriction.* Free Radic Biol. Med, 21:5, 651-68, 1996.

Yu, H., Oho, T., Tagomori, S., Morioka, T. *Anticarcinogenic effects of green tea.* Fukuoka Igaku Zasshi, Apr, 83:4, 174-80, 1992.

Zorgniotti, A.W., Lizza, E.F. *Effects of large doses of nitric oxide precursor, L-arginine on erectile disfunction.* Int J Impotence Res 6:33-36,1994.

INDEX

A

B

C

D

H

I

L

M

N

O

P

R

S

T

U

V

W

Y

Z